INFECTIONS AND
ARTHRITIS

NEW
CLINICAL
APPLICATIONS
RHEUMATOLOGY

INFECTIONS AND ARTHRITIS

Editors

JOHN J CALABRO†
MD, FACP
Professor of Medicine and Pediatrics
University of Massachusetts Medical School
Director of Rheumatology
Saint Vincent Hospital
Worcester, Massachusetts, USA

W CARSON DICK
MD (Glas.), MBChB, FRCP (Lond.)
Department of Rheumatology
Royal Victoria Infirmary
Newcastle upon Tyne
NE1 4LP, UK

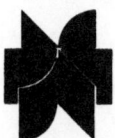

KLUWER ACADEMIC PUBLISHERS
DORDRECHT / BOSTON / LONDON

Distributors

for the United States and Canada: Kluwer Academic Publishers, PO Box 358, Accord Station, Hingham, MA 02018–0358, USA
for all other countries: Kluwer Academic Publishers Group, Distribution Center, PO Box 322, 3300 AH Dordrecht, The Netherlands

British Library Cataloguing in Publication Data

Infections and arthritis
  1. Man. Arthritis. Aetiology
  I. Calabro, John J.   II. Dick, W. Carson (William
  Carson)   III. Series
  616.7′22071

  ISBN-13: 978-94-010-6867-3   e-ISBN-13: 978-94-009-0845-1
  DOI: 10.1007/978-94-009-0845-1

Copyright

Published in the United Kingdom by Kluwer Academic Publishers, PO Box 55, Lancaster, UK.

Kluwer Academic Publishers BV incorporates the publishing programmes of D. Reidel, Martinus Nijhoff, Dr W. Junk and MTP Press.

CONTENTS

CONTENTS

LIST OF CONTRIBUTORS

S. L. Atkin
Department of Rheumatology
University of Newcastle upon
  Tyne Medical School
Royal Victoria Infirmary
Newcastle upon Tyne
UK

I. N. Bird
Department of Pathology
University of Bristol
The Medical School
University Walk
Bristol
UK

P. T. Dawes
Staffordshire Rheumatology
  Centre
Haywood Hospital, High Lane
Burslem
Stoke on Trent
UK

F. S. di Giovine
Department of Medicine
Rheumatic Diseases Unit

University of Edinburgh
Northern General Hospital
Edinburgh
UK

G. W. Duff
Department of Medicine
Rheumatic Diseases Unit
University of Edinburgh
Northern General Hospital
Edinburgh
UK

J. A. Goodacre
Department of Medicine
  (Rheumatology)
Catherine Cookson Building
The Medical School
Newcastle upon Tyne
UK

P. N. Platt
Department of Rheumatology
University of Newcastle upon
  Tyne Medical School
Royal Victoria Infirmary
Newcastle upon Tyne UK

T. P. Sheeran
Staffordshire Rheumatology
  Centre
Haywood Hospital
High Lane
Burslem
Stoke on Trent
UK

J. A. Symons
Department of Medicine
Rheumatic Diseases Unit
University of Edinburgh
Northern General Hospital
Edinburgh
UK

P. W. Thompson
Bone and Joint Research Unit
The London Hospital Medical
  College
Turner Street
London E1
UK

D. Walker
Department of Medicine
University of Newcastle upon
  Tyne Medical School
Royal Victoria Infirmary
Newcastle upon Tyne
UK

D. J. Walker
Department of Rheumatology
University of Newcastle upon
  Tyne Medical School
Royal Victoria Infirmary
Newcastle upon Tyne
UK

A. D. Woolf
Royal Cornwall Hospital
  (City)
Infirmary Hill
Truro
Cornwall
UK

SERIES EDITOR'S FOREWORD

The relationship between infection and arthritis has occupied the attention of everybody throughout the history of investigative rheumatology, no less today than formerly[1]. The present issue is a compilation of essays reflecting some of the facets of this particular diamond and I am especially grateful to authors and publishers alike in the unusual and tragic circumstances which attended its preparation.

We were all stunned and saddened by the untimely death of Professor John Calabro which deprived us of a good friend and wise counsellor as well as a much esteemed professional colleague. Prof. Calabro's contribution to medicine was considerable, spanning highly individual, exemplary and caring clinical management, enthusiastic charismatic teaching at all levels and major contributions to research particularly in the field of juvenile arthritis. As with Robert Burns, whose works John knew, "when will we see his like again?". A personal sadness is that I was looking forward to welcoming John and his wife to "Geordieland". There is a strong tradition of the highest level of competitive ballroom dancing here and John was looking forward to visiting us and demonstrating the considerable skills which he and his wife displayed in this arena. To his wife and family we all extend our heartfelt condolences.

W. CARSON DICK

1. Atkin, S., Walker, D., Mander, M., Malcolm, A. and Dick, W. Carson. (1988). Observation on the causes of rheumatoid arthritis. *Br. J. Rheumatol.,* **27** (Suppl. 2), 173–175

1

THE RED HOT JOINT – ACUTE MONOARTHRITIS

P. N. Platt

INTRODUCTION AND DIFFERENTIAL DIAGNOSIS

The red hot joint or acute monoarthritis is one of the most important and satisfying diagnostic challenges in rheumatology. The rapid and accurate diagnosis of this problem can prevent potential severe and permanent joint damage and occasionally death. As such, acute monoarthritis must be treated as a medical emergency.

A wide range of conditions can produce acute monoarthritis which, for the purposes of this chapter, is defined as a monoarthritis with significant features of inflammation of less than 14 days duration. Many of the causes of acute monoarthritis, including gout, calcium pyrophosphate arthropathy, reactive arthritis and septic arthritis, are also frequent causes of oligoarthritis.

The satisfaction in dealing with patients with monoarthritis comes not only from the knowledge of potential benefit to the patient but also from the application of clinical skills, practical skills and laboratory investigations leading to a precise diagnosis in a high proportion of cases[1]. The clinical skills required are those which are central to good medical practice, i.e. accurate and informed history taking and careful medical examination. The principal practical skill required is the ability to aspirate joints. Many of the laboratory skills required should be available directly to the clinician, including polarizing light microscopy and the ability to produce appropriately stained microscope slides.

1

The differential diagnosis of acute monoarthritis or oligoarthritis includes a wide range of conditions. The principal ones are classified in Table 1.1.

The list given in Table 1.1 is not exhaustive. Other conditions have been reported to cause acute monoarthritis but are very infrequent causes, emphasizing the wide range of conditions that may have to be considered.

TABLE 1.1   Differential diagnosis of acute monoarthritis

1. Acute bacterial infections	
2. Crystal-induced diseases	– Gout
	– Calcium pyrophosphate arthropathy
	– Calcium hydroxyapatite arthropathy
3. Trauma	
4. Spontaneous haemarthrosis	– Clotting disorders
	– Anticoagulants
	– Local synovial abnormalities e.g. PVNS
5. Reactive arthritis	
6. Acute osteomyelitis close to a joint	
7. Local soft tissue lesion	– Infection
	– Crystal induced
	– Trauma
8. Initial phase of a chronic disorder	– Rheumatoid arthritis
	– Psoriatic arthritis
	– Ankylosing spondylitis
	– Osteoarthritis
	– SLE, PAN, etc.

PVNS = pigmented villonodular synovitis

HISTORY

It is important to take a detailed and accurate history. A knowledge of potential differential diagnoses allows appropriate lines of questioning to be followed. Unstructured questions and the failure to ask specific direct questions about, for example, urethritis and sexual contacts may lead to a diagnostic failure.

The patient should be questioned about trauma at an early stage of the history taking. Series of cases of monoarthritis differ considerably in the proportion in which the cause was trauma. This is dependent on the source of patients and the amount of prior screening of the patient. In most rheumatological series, the incidence of trauma is low. If a history of trauma is elicited, it is important to try to establish its significance. Many patients with gout or acute calcium pyrophosphate arthropathy describe trauma to the affected joint a few days before the onset of monoarthritis. Less specifically, many patients who develop monoarthritis will have remembered a recent and otherwise unmemorable episode of minor everyday trauma to which they attribute significance. A history of recent trauma, unless major, should not be accepted as the cause of acute monoarthritis to the exclusion of further investigation. A history of an acute monoarthritis starting four to seven days after physical stress, such as surgery, is suggestive of gout or calcium pyrophosphate arthropathy.

It is important to establish the mode of onset of the acute mono-arthritis. The history of a patient being awakened by acute pain and inflammation in the great toe is very suggestive of gout. The sudden onset of pain when twisting the knee is suggestive of a mechanical cause. If the affected joint is only one of a number of joints affected to a lesser degree, or that have been affected in the immediate past, it increases the likelihood of one of the causes of polyarthritis presenting in an atypical way. These include reactive arthritides, seronegative spondarthritides, rheumatoid arthritis, etc.

Questioning about the quality of pain may be helpful, pain at rest and stiffness being suggestive of an inflammatory cause. Pain may also be referred, the best example being the pain from disease in the hip being felt in the knee. A history of systemic illness, including shivering, rigors and pyrexia, may be obtained, particularly in those with septic arthritis. A history of influenza 10–14 days prior to the onset of acute monoarthritis is suggestive of staphylococcal infection.

A detailed history is particularly important in cases of reactive arthritis and must include any episodes of diarrhoeal illness, however minor, sexual contacts, urethritis, rashes and conjunctivitis. Urethritis may appear as part of the complex of reactive arthritis associated with

3

bowel organism-triggered disease and should not be assumed to be evidence of sexually transmitted disease. The speed and frequency of modern travel means that infections acquired abroad may be imported as a cause of monoarthritis. Therefore, a history of recent foreign travel and any insect bites may be relevant.

A history of previous episodes of acute monoarthritis may be important. Recurrent attacks of podagra are strongly suggestive, but not diagnostic, of gout. Recurrent episodes involving knees and wrists are suggestive of calcium pyrophosphate arthropathy. A history of recent intra-articular injections raises the possibility of iatrogenic infection.

A number of the conditions causing acute monoarthritis have a familial tendency and therefore a family history of gout, ankylosing spondylitis, rheumatoid arthritis, hyperlipidaemia, etc. may be important.

Drugs can modify the clinical features of an acute monoarthritis. Knowledge of the patient's consumption of non-steroidal anti-inflammatory drugs (NSAIDs), including aspirin, corticosteroids and antibiotics, is important. NSAIDs and corticosteroids are potent anti-inflammatory agents which are capable of negating many of the inflammatory features of an acute monoarthritis. The inflammatory features of even septic arthritis will 'respond' very well to NSAIDs with potentially dire consequences. It is this masking of symptoms by anti-inflammatory agents which can make the diagnosis of septic arthritis in conditions such as rheumatoid arthritis very difficult. It is not recommended that anti-inflammatory agents are used in the treatment of patients with an acute monoarthritis until a firm diagnosis has been made. This is also true of antibiotics where casual use of antibiotics can modify the clinical picture and render accurate diagnosis impossible. An analogy with the use of antibiotics in subacute bacterial endocarditis is apt.

EXAMINATION

The examination of a patient with acute monoarthritis can be considered in two parts: examination of the appropriate joint or peri-articular structures in detail and a general medical examination of

4

the patient. Care in examination and concern to avoid unnecessary discomfort to the patient is frequently repaid in ability to examine the patient in more detail. If a painful but important procedure is required, leave it to the end of the examination. The fact that the patient is very unwilling to allow you to examine a joint can be a useful sign of marked inflammation.

On inspection, it is important to note the colour of the affected joint. The genuinely bright red joint is evidence of intense inflammation and favours the most inflammatory conditions, such as bacterial infection or crystal-induced disease. A dark red or purple discoloration of the joint may be a feature of any of the inflammatory conditions. Evidence of trauma in terms of bruising or puncture marks should be sought. As well as changes in colour, the joint and periarticular area often has an increased temperature compared with surrounding areas.

Swelling of a joint may be due to effusion, soft tissue swelling or bony enlargement. Due to the acute nature of the problem, it is unlikely that bony enlargement is directly relevant although it may be a sign of preceding problems. It is important to identify the source of the swelling anatomically. The distinction between swelling arising from the joint or from periarticular structures is significant, as is the difference between an effusion and fluid in periarticular structures, such as bursi or a Baker's cyst.

The localization of tenderness is important. If the process is affecting the joint itself, it should be tender over the whole of the joint margins. Localization of tenderness to a particular point suggests a periarticular structure rather than the joint itself. It is then important to identify the structure or structures involved. If tenderness is localized to tendinous insertion into bone, it suggests an enthesopathy typical of the reactive arthritides and seronegative spondarthritides. Acute inflammation in bursi, due to a number of causes, including trauma, infection and crystal-induced diseases, may mimic acute monoarthritis. Accurate localization of the problem should be the first step in diagnosis.

Occasionally, a cellulitis occurring close to a joint may be difficult to distinguish from acute monoarthritis. In the case of gout and septic arthritis, there may be a significant cellulitic reaction associated with the affected joint. One mechanism by which this occurs is rupture of a joint capsule. This mechanism is applicable to any joint in which there is rapid formation of an effusion. It is best recognized in the

5

knee with the formation and rupture of a Baker's cyst. Normal synovial fluid released into soft tissues produces little reaction. However, if fluid from an actively inflamed joint, particularly a septic joint, is released into soft tissue, then a dramatic cellulitic reaction is provoked. This may even overshadow the original problem. The direction in which the fluid tends to track is dependent on the posture of the patient. In the case of a knee joint of a mobile patient, the fluid will normally track down into the calf. If the rupture occurs at a time when the patient is already on bed rest, which reduces the likelihood of the occurrence, the fluid may track into the thigh.

It is important to assess whether there is any evidence of tenderness over bone. An acute osteomyelitis close to a joint can present as an apparent acute monoarthritis including the presence of a sympathetic effusion[2]. It is also important to detect at an early stage the presence of osteomyelitis in periarticular bone secondary to a primary septic arthritis as this may have implications for treatment.

The range of movement in the affected joint is important. In an acutely inflamed joint, there may be no movement in any direction, the limitation of movement being due to a combination of pain and muscle spasm. In periarticular problems, there is often maintenance of movement until the particular structure is brought into play.

On general examination, the presence of pyrexia may be important but cannot be assumed to be due to infection. Patients with severe attacks of gout are frequently pyrexial[3], the pyrexia presumably being mediated through the release of interleukin-1.

Lymphadenopathy in the areas draining an inflamed joint is to be expected. However, generalized lymphadenopathy may suggest an underlying process leading to an immune compromised state predisposing to infection.

The skin should be examined for rashes, ulcers, pustules, infarcts, needle marks, suggesting iv drug abuse, tophi, xanthomata, etc. As listed above, a wide range of dermatological markers may be important in the differential diagnosis of acute monoarthritis. Many are important clues to an infective or reactive aetiology. The presence of ulceration or other septic focus may provide clues to the portal of entry of an infection. The range of infective organisms capable of causing septic arthritis or a reactive arthritis is extensive and, hence, the number of possible dermatological manifestations is too great to record here in detail. Some of the common or characteristic manifestations include: pustular lesions and infarcts in gonococcal septicaemia, vasculitic infarcts in staphylococcal septicaemia, vasculitic lesions in Henoch–Schönlein purpura, keratoderma blennorrhagica and balanitis in Reiter's syndrome. Non-infective skin lesions include tophaceous deposits. Although these are a late feature in primary gout they may be an early or even presenting feature in diuretic-induced gout[4]. Xanthomata raise the possibility of hyperlipidaemia, which is associated with a number of patterns of arthropathy, including a monoarthritis[5].

A detailed general examination of all systems is required, for example acute monoarthritis is a recognized presentation of subacute bacterial endocarditis. Conjunctivitis and uveitis are features of reactive arthritis.

EXAMINATION OF SYNOVIAL FLUID

The aspiration of a joint to obtain a sample of synovial fluid for examination is central to the management of acute monoarthritis. Joint aspiration is a safe procedure. The potential benefits exceed the possible drawbacks in the vast majority of cases. The main contraindications occur when the pathology is extra-articular. If the problem is a cellulitis close to a joint, but the joint is felt to be normal on clinical grounds, it may be wiser not to attempt to aspirate the joint through the cellulitis for fear of introducing infection into the joint. Anticoagulation is not a significant contraindication to aspiration. Good technique and a 21 gauge needle should produce no significant trauma.

Small amounts of synovial fluid may be valuable in making a diagnosis. Even the contents of the aspirating needle can be expelled and used to produce a slide for microscopy. The priorities are making slides and culture. If no fluid is obtained and septic arthritis is suspected the joint should be irrigated with saline and the aspirate sent for culture.

TABLE 1.2   Examination of synovial fluid

---

1. General description
2. Culture
3. White cell count
4. Conventional light microscopy
5. Polarizing light microscopy
6. Special tests

General description

Normal synovial fluid is clear and colourless or pale yellow. The turbidity of abnormal synovial fluid increases as the white cell count increases. This correlates roughly with the degree of inflammation present. Turbid synovial fluid can, however, be due to the presence of large quantities of crystals, lipids, fibrin or cartilage fragments. Rice bodies, so called because of their resemblance to polished rice, occur in inflammatory fluids, particularly from septic arthritis. They are formed by microinfarction of synovial villi[6].

The presence of blood in the aspirate may indicate a traumatic tap or one of the true causes of haemarthrosis. These include: trauma, synovial vessel abnormalities and pigmented villonodular synovitis and bleeding disorders, including haemophilia, thrombocytopenia and anticoagulants. In some cases, no obvious cause of bleeding is found. A traumatic tap can normally be distinguished as the blood is not evenly distributed and may clot locally. Normally synovial fluid does not clot due to the absence of fibrinogen and several clotting factors. However, pathological synovial fluid may clot, the size of the clot being roughly proportional to the degree of inflammation[7].

Culture of synovial fluid

It should be a routine procedure to culture the synovial fluid from all cases of acute monoarthritis even though the diagnosis appears obvious. If possible, avoid contaminating the synovial fluid sample with local anaesthetic.

8

When adequate volumes of synovial fluid are obtained, they should be divided as follows: 5–10 ml in a sterile container for culture and antibiotic sensitivity; 4 ml into an EDTA tube for total white cell counts and differential counts; a small volume to make several slides. The remainder should be stored at 4°C for further use depending on preliminary findings. It is important that the sterile container used for the synovial fluid sample is previously unused. Recycled containers have been found to contain dead bacteria which may cause diagnostic difficulties on Gram-stained slides[8]. If there is any difficulty in transporting the samples to the laboratory, it is wise to inoculate a small volume of synovial fluid into 'blood culture bottles'. A greater success rate for the isolation of organisms can be achieved if there is close co-operation with the bacteriology department for handling of samples and appropriate cultures. Synovial fluid antibiotic levels measured on repeated aspirations can help to ensure adequate antibiotic levels.

White cell counts

White cell counts can be performed either with a Coulter counter or with a haemocytometer and microscope. Very viscous samples of synovial fluid may cause technical difficulties with a Coulter counter because of the high viscosity. Normal synovial fluid contains less than 0.5×10^9 cells per litre. Pathological fluids can be categorized as non-inflammatory (0.5×10^9 to 5×10^9 per litre), inflammatory (5×10^9 to 50×10^9 per litre) and septic (greater than 50×10^9 per litre). In one large series, the cell counts in septic arthritis were greater than 50×10^9 cells per litre in 70% of cases[9]. The cases of septic arthritis with white cell counts below 50×10^9 comprised two groups: those with relatively mild disease, often gonococcal, and a second group with a high mortality who appeared unable to mount a normal leukocytosis. Gout and calcium pyrophosphate arthropathy occasionally show white cell counts above 50×10^9 per litre. The possibility of coexisting infection with these conditions is well recognized[10,11].

Conventional light microscopy

Fresh synovial fluid should be examined under the microscope as soon as possible to minimize artefacts. Initially, the slide should be scanned using a low-power lens to detect the presence of cells, cartilage fragments and fibrin clots. Cytoplasmic inclusions can be seen in some polymorphonuclear leukocytes. These are best seen using phase contrast microscopy or the partial phase effect produced by increasing the distance of the condenser from the slide. Their presence has been reported in rheumatoid arthritis, gout, calcium pyrophosphate arthropathy and infection[12]. The so-called Reiter's cells[13], macrophages that have phagocytosed polymorphs, have not proved to be specific for that condition[14]. Fat cells and bone spicules are occasionally seen and are indicative of trauma and possible intra-articular fracture.

Differential white cell counts require the use of stained preparations for accurate identification. A few drops of methylene blue added to the synovial fluid is helpful but better results are obtained by the use of a dried smear of synovial fluid stained with Wright's stain. Details of the method are contained in reference[12]. In synovial fluids from non-inflammatory conditions, mononuclear cells predominate. As the cell counts increase, the polymorphonuclear leucocyte becomes the predominant cell. Monocytosis has been described in patients with acute arthritis associated with virus infections, particularly hepatitis B and rubella[15].

The use of Gram's stain may provide a rapid diagnosis in a case of suspected septic arthritis and allow the use of more specific antibiotic treatment. A Gram stain showing no bacteria does not exclude infection. It may be difficult to detect Gram-negative bacteria due to the background of cells and debris. Positive smears for Gram-negative bacteria were found in only 50% of culture-proven cases in one series[16]. False positive results may be produced by irregular staining of clots producing an appearance similar to clumps of Gram-positive cocci.

Polarizing light microscopy

The use of polarizing light microscopy has enhanced the ability of a clinician to make an accurate diagnosis in cases of acute monoarthritis due to crystal-induced diseases. Crystalline material is highlighted on a polarizing light microscope due to the property of crystals of birefringence. Accurate identification of small crystals requires the use of a purpose-built polarizing light microscope. Meaningful results can be obtained with a conventional light microscope if fitted with polarizing lenses, particularly if a compensator can also be fitted between the specimen and the analyser. Detailed accounts of the physics of polarizing light microscopy are available[17],[12]. Polarizing light microscopy is a powerful technique but prone to form artefacts in the hands of the inexperienced or unwary.

It is important that the microscope, slides and coverslips are kept dust free. Also it is important to select 'clean' slides. Many new slides are covered with birefringent material which shows up under the polarizing light microscope and makes the identification of small crystals difficult. Synovial fluid samples should be examined as soon as possible with the polarizing light microscope as storage may lead to the artefactual formation of crystals. Brushite crystals, occurring as large positively birefringent crystals frequently arranged in a star, have been described in this context as have urate crystals[18]. If the slide is not to be examined immediately, it is important to seal the edge of the coverslip with a sealant to prevent drying and the formation of artefacts. It is possible to examine dried slides stained with Wright's stain although this does reduce the diagnostic yield[19].

Polarizing light microscopy should be commenced with a low-power lens and the polarizing lens set crossed to produce a dark background. In this mode, crystalline material will show up as bright objects against the dark background. When birefringent material has been identified, more detailed observation using the compensator and a high-power lens is required. Crystals have predominantly sharp, straight, clearly defined edges in contrast to the indistinct forms of many artefacts. Although extracellular crystals may be of significance, intracellular crystals are more likely to be a genuine finding unless crystalline artefacts, such as lithium heparin, were introduced before the slide was made.

11

Monosodium urate crystals (MSU) and gout

MSU crystals are typically needle-shaped, negatively birefringent crystals which are diagnostic of gout. In practical terms, negatively birefringent crystals are crystals that appear yellow when the long axis of the crystal is parallel to the axis of the polarizing light microscope. The axis is normally marked by the compensator. They are typically 2–20 μm in length and intracellular, or at least attached to polymorphonuclear leucocytes. The absence of MSU crystals does not exclude a diagnosis of gout but the finding of a single crystal is significant. In cases where crystals are absent in an otherwise typical attack of gout, it is worthwhile reaspirating the joint 24 h later when crystals will often be found.

Calcium pyrophosphate crystals (CPPD) and calcium pyrophosphate arthropathy

CPPD crystals are diagnostic of calcium pyrophosphate arthropathy or pseudogout. They are variable in size and shape but are normally in the range of 1–10 μm, smaller crystals being beyond the resolution of light microscopy. The classical description is of a rhomboid shape, often with a chip taken out of one corner. They are usually weakly positively birefringent. In some cases, the crystals appear square and it is difficult to distinguish the long axis and hence its optical axis. The number of crystals seen in very variable as is their intra- or extracellular location. Fibrin clots should be examined if present, as CPPD crystals are frequently found entangled in them. It may be difficult to distinguish small extracellular CPPD crystals from artefacts and it is wise to under- rather than over-diagnose if not sure.

Cholesterol crystals

There are recognized readily by their large size, 10–100 μm, and their appearance as stacked rectangular or rhomboid plates. They have been described in a number of hyperlipoproteinaemias and rheumatoid arthritis[20,21].

Other crystal types

Calcium hydroxyapatite crystals cannot be identified accurately by polarizing light microscopy but their presence can be inferred by small weakly birefringent masses of material with an appearance like stacked coins. The use of alizarin red stain has been suggested as a method of detecting calcium hydroxyapatite crystals[22] but it is not specific and prone to artefact. Brushite crystals, large strongly positively birefringent crystals, have been reported[23] but may be artefactual[18]. The depot forms of several local steroid preparations are crystalline in form and may persist for some time after injection. When seen in synovial fluid, they are normally present in large numbers, variable in size and very optically active. Calcium oxalate crystals, recognized by their characteristic pyramidal shape have been reported in effusions in patients on maintenance haemodialysis[24].

Other tests on synovial fluid

A low synovial fluid glucose, when compared with a paired serum sample, is said to suggest infection. This is non-specific and purely a function of a high white cell number and provides no evidence beyond a white cell count. Protein and complement levels are non-specific and rarely of diagnostic significance. Rheumatoid factors and antinuclear factors produce more difficulty in interpretation than diagnostic help[1].

OTHER INVESTIGATIONS

Radiology

An X-ray film of affected and contralateral joints are an essential part of the investigation of a patient with acute monoarthritis. After synovial fluid examination, it is the investigation most likely to produce a diagnosis[1]. Many of the films taken will be normal apart from changes in soft tissue swelling, non-specific oedema and effusion. However, they are still of importance as they provide a baseline for further comparison. Calcification of articular cartilage, chondro-calcinosis, may be due to the deposition of a range of calcium

13

salts. The best recognized and most common is CPPD in calcium pyrophosphate arthropathy. Calcium hydroxyapatite and brushite have also been reported although the significance of brushite is not clear. Calcium oxalate crystals producing chondrocalcinosis has been reported in haemodialysis patients[24]. Soft tissue calcification in periarticular structures may be of significance and is almost invariably due to calcium hydroxyapatite crystals. Calcific supraspinatus tendinitis is the best recognized of the calcific periarticular syndromes. It is frequently misdiagnosed as an acute monoarthritis because of the intense inflammation induced by the release of the calcium hydroxyapatite crystals. Synovial calcification suggests osteochondromatosis or pigmented villonodular synovitis.

The time course of radiological change in bone is such that any boney changes seen, apart from fractures, must pre-date the symptoms of acute monoarthritis. Radio-isotope scanning with either technetium or gallium is not normally of sufficient specificity to be diagnostic. It may provide evidence of acute osteomyelitis prior to conventional radiology and may identify early disease at sites other than the presenting joint.

Blood tests

No single haematological, biochemical or serological investigation can be considered diagnostic. White cell counts are elevated in most, but not all, cases of septic arthritis and some cases of gout. A normal white cell count in septic arthritis may be indicative of failure to respond normally and a poor prognosis. Hyperuricaemia is too common for uric acid levels to be of value in the diagnosis of gout. Although a normal level makes a diagnosis of gout unlikely, it does not exclude it.

Autoantibodies and complement levels are non-specific, and, in one series of 59 patients with acute monoarthritis, they were not of diagnostic significance[1]. If a reactive or viral arthritis is suspected, serological and viral titres may be informative.

14

Bacteriological cultures

In addition to the routine culture of synovial fluid samples, swabs from skin lesions, urethra and vagina may be indicated. If septic arthritis is suspected blood cultures should be taken.

Arthroscopy

In cases of acute monoarthritis which have proved resistant to diagnosis and persistent, arthroscopy offers increased diagnostic possibilities by direct visualization and synovial biopsy for culture and histology. Direct visualization makes the technique superior to blind needle biopsy in obtaining tissue for histology.

CONCLUSIONS

A wide range of conditions are capable of producing acute mono-arthritis and are amenable to diagnosis. Some cases of acute mono-arthritis remain resistant to diagnosis, but, in many instances, these have a good prognosis with symptoms resolving, the aetiology of their monoarthritis remaining obscure. The speed of diagnosis is important, particularly in cases of septic arthritis[25] where a delay of 24 hours may alter the prognosis significantly. With accurate early diagnosis and appropriate treatment, the prognosis for the vast majority of patients is excellent.

REFERENCES

1. Freed, J. F., Nies, K. M., Boyer, R. S. and Louie, J. S. (1980). Acute monoarticular arthritis – a diagnostic approach. *J. Am. Med. Assoc.*, **243**, 2314–2316
2. Platt, P. N. and Griffiths, I. D. (1984). Pyrogenic osteomyelitis presenting as an acute sterile arthropathy. *Ann. Rheum. Dis.*, **43**, 607–609
3. Woolf, A. D., Nouri, A. M. E., Woo, P., Richter, M. B., Panayi, G. S. and Gibson, T. (1985). Interleukin-1 and the acute phase response in acute crystal synovitis. *Br. J. Rheum.*, **24** (suppl. 1), 203–208
4. Platt, P. N. and Dick, W. C. (1985) Diuretic induced gout – The beginnings of an epidemic. *Practitioner*, **229**, 282–284

5. Rooney, P. N., Dallantype, D. and Buchanan, W. W. (1975). Disorders of the locomotor system associated with lipid metabolism and lipoidoses. *Clin. Rheum. Dis.*, **1**, 163–194

6. Cheung, H. S., Ryan, L., Kozin, F. and McCarty, D. J. (1980). Synovial origins of rice bodies in joint fluid. *Arth. Rheum.*, **23**, 72–76

7. Ropes, M. W. and Bauer, W. (1953). *Synovial Fluid Changes in Joint Disease.* (Cambridge, MA: Harvard University Press)

8. Freeman, R. and Jones, M. R. (1983). Microbiology. In Jeffrey, M. S. and Dick, W. C. (eds.) *Clin. Rheum. Dis.*, **9**, 3–26

9. Krey, P. R. and Bailen, D. A. (1979). Synovial fluid leucocytosis – a study of extremes. *Am. J. Med.*, **67**, 436–442

10. Smith, R. J. and Phelps, I. (1972) Septic arthritis, gout, pseudogout and osteoarthritis in the knee of a patient with multiple myeloma. *Arthritis Rheum.*, **15**, 89–96

11. Jarrett, M. P. and Grayzel, A. I. (1980). Simultaneous gout, pseudogout and septic arthritis. *Arth. Rheum.*, **23**, 128–129

12. Platt, P. N. (1983). Examination of synovial fluid. In Jeffrey, M. S. and Dick, W. C. (eds. *Clin. Rheum. Dis.*, **9**, 51–67

13. Pekin, T. J., Maknin, T. I. and Zvaiffler, N. J. (1967). Unusual synovial fluid findings in Reiter's syndrome. *Ann. Int. Med.*, **66**, 677–684

14. Mowat, A. G., Spriggs, A. and Boddington, H. (1978). The diagnostic value of 'Reiter's cells'. *Ann. Rheum. Dis.*, **37**, 489

15. Schmid, F. R. (1981). Approach to monoarticular arthritis. In Kelley, W. N., Harris, E. D., Ruddy, S. and Sledge, C. B. (eds.) *Textbook of Rheumatology*, pp. 384–92. (Philadelphia: W. B. Saunders)

16. Goldenberg, D. L., Brandt, K. D., Cathcart, E. S. and Cohen, A. S. (1974). Acute arthritis caused by Gram negative bacilli: a clinical characterisation. *Medicine*, **53**, 197–208

17. Fagan, T. J. and Lidsky, M. D. (1974). Compensated polarising light microscopy using cellophane adhesive tape. *Arthritis Rheum.*, **17**, 256–262

18. Dieppe. P. A. and Calvert, P. (1983). *Crystals and Joint Disease.* (London: Chapman and Hall)

19. Phelps, P., Steele, A. D. and McCarty, D. J. (1968). Compensated polarised light microscopy. *J. Am. Med. Assoc.*, **203**, 508–512

20. Zuckner, J., Uddin, J., Gautner, G. E. and Dorner, R. W. (1964). Cholesterol crystals in synovial fluid. *Ann. Intern. Med.*, **60**, 439–446

21. Pritzker, K. P. H., Fam, A. G., Omar, S. A. and Geryzbein, S. D. (1981). Experimental cholesterol crystal arthropathy. *J. Rheumatol.*, **8**, 281–290

22. Paul, H. and Reginato, A. J. (1980). Alizarin red staining as a screening test to detect calcium compounds in synovial fluid. *Arthritis Rheum*, **19**, 730

23. Gaucher, A., Faure, G., Netter, P. and Pourel, J. (1978). Single crystal identification of calcium hydrogen phosphate dihydrate in destructive arthropathies of chondrocalcinosis. *Eur. J. Rheum. Inflamm.*, **1**, 120–124

24. Hoffman, G. S., Schumacher, H. R., Paul, H., Cherian, V., Reed, R., Ramsay, A. G. and Frank, W. A. (1982). Calcium oxalate microcrystalline associated arthritis in end stage renal failure. *Ann. Intern. Med.*, **97**, 36–42

25. Broy, S. B. and Schmid, F. R. (1986). A comparison of medical drainage and surgical drainage in the initial treatment of infected joints. *Clin. Rheum. Dis.*, **12**, 501–523

2

THE RELATIONSHIP BETWEEN BACTERIA, RELATED ORGANISMS AND CHRONIC ARTHRITIS

P. T. DAWES and T. SHEERAN

INTRODUCTION

There is a historical causative association between arthritis and infection. This has now been firmly established as an aetiological relationship following advances in the fields of microbiology, immunogenetics and clinical rhematology. Astute observation and belief in an infective cause for arthritis has provided rheumatologists with many of the current anti-arthritic drugs. At the end of the last century, gold was shown to inhibit growth of tubercle bacilli and Forestier, assuming tuberculosis and rheumatoid shared a common aetiology, showed it to be effective for arthritis[1]. Gold also inhibits mycoplasma, which have also been implicated in causing rheumatoid arthritis[2]. Sulphasalazine was developed in the belief that rheumatoid arthritis was infective in origin[3]. Following initially disappointing trials, it has now been shown to be effective in both ankylosing spondylitis[4] and rheumatoid arthritis[5]. In rheumatoid arthritis, it is the bacteriostatic sulphapyridine that is the active moiety[6]. The sulphones, dapsone[7] and sulphamethoxazole[8] are also effective in rheumatoid arthritis. There are many other drugs, i.e. chloroquine, levamisole, metronidazole, clotrimazole, rifampicin, derived for infective conditions, which have been used with variable success in the treatment of rheumatoid arthritis. With our better understanding, it is foreseen

17

that there will be a more rational approach to diagnosis and management of many rheumatic diseases. In this chapter, we have attempted to encompass the many facets relating infection to chronic arthritis. We hope this is conveyed with some enthusiasm to stimulate the reader's perception of this important topic.

BACTERIAL INFECTION IN PATIENTS WITH ESTABLISHED ARTHRITIS

Reduced mobility, reduced nutrition, end organ damage, the presence of damaged joints and prostheses and drug treatment, including non-steroidal anti-inflammatory drugs[9], all predispose the chronic arthritic to infection. In rheumatoid arthritis and systemic lupus erythematosis, there are also impaired host defence mechanisms associated with the disease.

Rheumatoid arthritis

Infection may contribute to morbidity and mortality in rheumatoid arthritis[10], increasingly since the use of immunosuppressive agents[11]. Pulmonary and renal tract infection, skin sepsis and septic arthritis are most common[12,13]. Rheumatoid patients with Felty's syndrome are particularly predisposed, being a specific subset of rheumatoid arthritis strongly associated[14] with DRW4, sero-positivity for IgM rheumatoid factor, often with a positive antinuclear factor. Although joint damage may be severe, inflammatory synovitis is often clinically inactive. Neutropenia is the cardinal defect in Felty's syndrome and can occur in rheumatoid without the other features. Neutropenia may even precede the signs of arthritis[15,16]. Although neutropenic rheumatoid patients are predisposed to infection[11], the peripheral blood neutrophil count correlates poorly with the number and severity of infective episodes[17] and patients can remain infection free for many years[18]. Infections are often due to common organisms[19]. During infection, the neutrophil count may return to normal but is seldom elevated. The bone marrow picture varies from normal to myeloid hyperplasia with maturation arrest; rarely does it show depression of myeloid activity[17]. A moderate anaemia, due to shortened red blood cell survival, and thrombocytopenia occur. There are two basic mechanisms contributing to the pathogenesis of rheumatoid neutropenia:

(1) Increased removal – laden with complexes[20,21], neutrophils are sequestrated in the spleen[22]. Neutrophil antibodies often occurring in antinuclear factor positive individuals also reduce survival time[23,24].

(2) Reduced proportion – reduced neutrophil reserves result from an inhibition of maturation[25,26], possibly mediated by T suppressor cells[27].

As well as neutropenia there is also neutrophil dysfunction due to impaired chemotaxis and phagocytosis[28–31]. Hypocomplementaemia[24], IgA deficiency and hypogammaglobulinaemia may also be important predisposing factors.

Systemic lupus erythematosus

The major cause of death in the presteroid era was infection and this is still the most likely cause of pyrexia in active disease[32]. Infections may relate to the relative deficiency of complement, important in bacterial killing. This lack of complement can result in large insoluble immune complexes which are not dispersed by the reticulo-endothelial system but still impair its function[33,34]. Infections can precipitate disease flares, and a rise in DNA antibodies and other immune parameters does not exclude infection. C-reactive protein is helpful in distinguishing between infection and active disease. It is marginally raised during a disease flare but very high if infection is present. In unwell patients, infection, including opportunistic infections, must be diligently sought. Often, treatment is commenced before the results of cultures are known.

ORGANISMS CAUSING CHRONIC ARTHRITIS

It is apparent that organisms induce different patterns of arthritis by a number of different mechanisms. For convenience we have examined the relationship between infection causing arthritis from four, frequently merging, viewpoints:

(a) Chronic arthritis due to an intra-articular organism.
(b) Chronic arthritis due to extra-articular organisms (reactive arthritis).
(c) Animal models that demonstrate a relationship between bacteria and arthritis.
(d) Speculative and unproven links between chronic arthritis and infection.

ARTHRITIS DUE TO BACTERIAL INVASION OF THE JOINT

Tuberculous arthritis

Both typical (*Mycobacterium tuberculosis, M. bovis*) and atypical (e.g. *M. kanasii, M. avium, M. fortuitum*) forms of tubercle bacillus are capable of causing a chronic granulomatous arthritis. Although atypical infection is rare and difficult to confirm, it is an important cause of chronic joint sepsis[35]. Between 1 and 2% of patients with tuberculosis have skeletal disease, only half of whom have active pulmonary disease, yet almost all are Mantoux test positive. Skeletal infection is classically in the thoracolumbar spine resulting in disc destruction, vertebral collapse and gibbous deformity. A paraspinal abscess is often present and can lead to cord compression. Unilateral sacroiliitis is often a diagnostic dilemma and tuberculosis is a well-recognized cause. Extraspinal disease often affects the hip, and, less frequently, the knee, ankle or wrist. Usually it is mono-articular and insidious in onset, with presence of sinus tracts arousing suspiscion. Aspiration of a tuberculous joint can show 'rice bodies', culture may reveal acid-fast bacilli but diagnosis often requires synovial biopsy. Musculoskeletal infection can also present as chronic tenosynovitis, bursitis or dactylitis, particularly in children. The risk of developing this infection and its unusual manifestations is increased in certain ethnic groups[36].

Pulmonary tuberculosis has been implicated in causing a reactive arthritis (Poncet's disease) which is said to have a temporal relationship to pulmonary disease activity[37,38]. This manifestation is rare and, as an entity, remains questionable. Arthritis due to leprosy is covered elsewhere.

20

Brucellosis

Brucellosis is a zoonosis affecting a wide range of animals, the strains
B. suis (pig), *B. melitensis* (sheep), *B. canis* (dog) and *B. abortus*
(cattle) being the main human pathogens. Bone and joint disease com-
plicates about 9% of brucella infections but varies depending on where
the infection is contracted and which organism is prevalent[39]. In many
countries, infection is being eradicated in animals and disease is seen
only after occupational exposure[40]. Diagnosis is difficult and, in skeletal brucellosis, cultures are frequently negative[41]; positive serology
may be crucial[42]. This can bedevil the clinician trying to establish a
diagnosis as the infection may cause either joint sepsis (often spinal
or sacroiliac) requiring antibiotics or a reactive arthritis and spondarthritis. It is wise to regard all patients as having active infection
requiring antibiotics even in the absence of positive cultures[43]. The
type of arthritis may be dictated by the interaction between HLA
status and the antigen differences between brucella strains[44]. *Brucella
melitensis* and *B. abortus* are both reported as causing reactive
disease[45–47]. *Brucella abortus* infection in HLA B27 + ve individuals is
reported as causing a chronic spondarthritis[48].

Whipple's disease

This is a rare multisystem disease, commoner in males. It is characterized by episodes of polyarthritis[49] which may precede the other
manifestations of disease and mimic many arthropathies. Weight loss,
diarrhoea, lymphadenopathy, skin pigmentation, pleuro-pericardial
and progressive CNS disease may all occur[50]. Patients are often
anaemic, with steatorrhoea, reduced xylose absorption and partial
villous atrophy on jejunal biopsy. The attacks of arthritis can be
palindromic and severe joint deformity is unusual. Some patients
develop sacroiliitis and spondarthritis[51,52] although the relationship
with HLA B27 is not clear[53]. The diagnosis rests on identification of
PAS (periodic acid Schiff stain) staining macrophages in synovium
or jejunum on light microscopy. Electron microscopy demonstrates
intracellular micro-organisms[54]. It is difficult to define the arthritis as
a reactive or a true infective disease as the organism has not been fully

21

characterized nor cultured *in vitro*[55]. It would seem that the organism is sensitive to antibiotics which improve the arthritis. This suggests direct infection within the joint is important. When establishing the diagnosis, multiple jejunal biopsies may be required to show PAS-positive macrophages as skip lesions occur.

Lyme disease

Lyme disease was first described in Lyme, Connecticut, USA but is now recognized as having a worldwide distribution[56]. It is a salutory lesson that recognition of this disease was initially made by parents who had observed a clustering of arthritis around the summer and autumn months.

Lyme disease was thought to be an autoimmune illness but discovery of the tick-borne spirochaete, *Borrelia burgdorferi*, has revealed its true nature. Initially thought to be a disease confined to joints, it is recognized as a multisystem disorder with cardiovascular, neurological and dermatological manifestations which mimic a 'connective tissue disease'[57].

In Europe, the infection[58] causes a different clinical picture with chronic skin and neurological problems predominating. This may reflect subtle differences in the spirochaete though cases of arthritis are now being recognized[59-62]. The infection is transmitted to humans following a bite from *Ixodes dammini*, other related ticks and possibly fleas from deer, mice and even household pets. Following the initial description of the arthritis[63], it became apparent that Lyme disease has three major stages[64].

Stage 1

Three to 32 days after a tick bite, a pruritic skin lesion resembling a red ring occurs around the thigh, groin or axilla. This is called erythema chronicum migrans. This initial rash is often followed by smaller annular lesions covering the whole body except for the palms and soles. During this phase constitutional upset with fever, malaise, cough, headaches, meningism, arthralgia, splenomegaly, lymphadenopathy

22

and conjunctivitis occurs. There is associated anaemia, elevated ESR and raised IgM levels. Urine examination can suggest a transient glomerulitis although serum creatinine remains normal. It is possible, by an Elisa technique, to demonstrate an IgM-specific antibody to the spirochaete which reaches a peak level between 3 and 6 weeks. The presence of IgM cryoglobulins may predict later complications of disease. The appearance of an IgG antibody is often associated[65] with stages 2 and 3.

Stage 2

Cardiac and neurological complications occur weeks to months after the initial infection. Diffuse myocardial and pericardial disease occurs with varying forms of atrioventricular conduction defects. A further 10% develop significant neurological disease due to a lymphocytic meningoencephalitis, with transient cranial nerve palsys (often facial) and motor/sensory neuropathies.

Stage 3

This final stage may occur either weeks or years after inoculation with the spirochaete. It is characterized by chronic joint, skin or neurological disease. The neurological disease manifests as demyelination and progressive dementia[66], skin involvement by a wide spectrum of conditions, i.e. acrodermatitis chronica atrophicans, lymphocytosis cutis benigna and even morphea[67].

Joint disease is characterized by two merging phases. Sixty per cent of patients develop intermittent episodes of a monoarticular/oligoarticular/migratory arthritis during early disease which may last from weeks to months[68]. The commonest joint affected is the knee and lack of marked synovial swelling helps to differentiate it from seronegative rheumatoid arthritis. About 10% of patients progress and develop a chronic arthritis with palpable synovitis. The chronic joint, skin and neurological manifestations often occur in patients possessing the histocompatability antigen, DR2[69]. Synovial fluid examination shows an inflammatory fluid with reduced C3 complement, immune complexes and cryoglobulins. Although radiological erosion is unusual, histologically there is pannus formation with cartilage damage. The one major histological difference from rheumatoid is demonstration of the organism in 25% of synovial biopsies. Treatment in the early stage with tetracycline, penicillin or erthyromycin[64] seems to prevent progression to the later stages. Parenteral penicillin may be required in these later stages and can be complicated by a Herxheimer reaction. Unfortunately, not all cases resolve with antibiotics alone and prednisolone and hydroxychloroquine have been used for the neurological and joint disease. This suggests an autonomous inflammatory stage in the absence of viable organisms. Immunologically, it is similar to other arthropathies with lymphocytic dysfunction important in causing the long-term sequelae[70,71].

Other spirochaetes

Congenital syphilis can cause recurrent joint effusions (Clutton's joints) and be confused with juvenile arthritis[72]. Secondary syphilis with rash and fever can present as arthritis[73]. Tertiary disease is also associated with a synovitis as well as neuropathic and gummatous joints. Spondylitis with spinal ankylosis, and periostitis are also manifestations of this disease. The treponema causing Yaws can give rise to similar articular manifestations.

Leptospira, including *L. icterohaemorrhagiae*, have been reported as causing arthritis[74-77].

Streptobacillus moniliformis

This aerobic Gram-negative bacillus is an inhabitant of mice and rats. Following a bite, patients develop recurrent fever (rat bite fever), headache, malaise, lymphadenopathy, splenomegaly, a desquamative rash occasionally with pustules and arthritis[78]. The arthritis is usually polyarticular, affecting large and small joints. The organism can be demonstrated in synovial fluid. Unless treated with penicillin and streptomycin, the arthritis can persist and produce permanent joint damage.

24

Mycoplasma

Mycoplasma are the smallest free-living organisms and, although lacking a true cell wall, they do have a membrane enclosing cytoplasm, DNA and RNA. There are three main families of mycoplasma, of which Mycoplasmataceae are the important human pathogens. Two forms of joint problem are seen. Firstly, a reactive form; patients with a mycoplasma pneumonia may develop arthralgia and myalgia, with symptoms lasting up to 12 months[79-81]. Also, ureaplasma are involved in causing urethritis and hence reactive arthritis[82,83]. Secondly, mycoplasma may invade the joint producing a septic arthritis and are an important cause of arthritis in patients with hypogammaglobulinaemia. These patients are already prone to a polyarthritis requiring gammaglobulin[84] but, if a septic joint develops, active exclusion and treatment of mycoplasma is required[85-87].

REACTIVE ARTHRITIS

In simplistic terms, this form of arthritis is the result of an interaction between a susceptible human genotype and an organism, i.e. soil + seed = arthritis. The arthritis is caused by extra-articular infection in the absence of viable intra-articular organisms[88,89]. Reactive arthritis is characterized by:

(1) An interval between the triggering infection and the onset of arthritis.
(2) Negative synovial fluid culture.
(3) No response to antibiotics.

Although many reactive arthropathies were once regarded as self-limiting diseases, there is now evidence that many patients develop persistent joint problems. Reactive arthritis can be split into two broad categories[90]. Firstly, non-HLA B27-related arthropathy. Secondly, HLA B27-related arthropathies which occur after an increasingly recognized number of infections. These patients often display similar clinical features, but unfortunately possession of HLA B27 is not diagnostic. It is likely that there are other unrecognized host factors[91].

25

Reactive arthritis not related to HLA B27

Rheumatic fever

It has been suggested that this represents a streptococcal-induced auto-immune disease. It follows infection with Group A β-haemolytic streptococci, an organism that has similar antigens to those found in muscle sarcolemma[92,93]. Antibody deposition occurs on heart valves[94] and increased titres are associated with extracardiac complications, including arthritis[95]. There would seem to be a genetic predisposition to rheumatic fever[95] which has not been shown to be HLA linked. Rheumatic fever, now rare in children in developed countries, is still seen in adults. The diagnosis may be missed as the cause of arthritis as the other clinical findings of carditis, chorea and skin lesions, are often absent[96]. The adult arthropathy is often a progressive symmetrical large joint disease with associated tenosynovitis. This often develops within a week of infection[97]. This contrasts with chronic rheumatic fever where recurrent attacks can produce a deformity similar to rheumatoid arthritis (Jaccoud's arthritis)[98].

Meningococcal arthritis

Arthritis is a recognized complication[99] in 2–10% of patients with meningococcal meningitis. However, arthralgia is more usual than arthritis, and affects the knee, wrist, elbow and ankle. Onset of the joint disease coincides with an urticarial or vasculitic rash[100] and occasionally episcleritis. These usually occur when the meningeal signs are resolving. Different forms of arthritis have been reported[101], including joint sepsis[102] and Reiter's syndromes[103]. In the majority, the arthritis, is due to deposition of IgM immune complexes with complement activation[104]. The immune complex is in response to a specific meningococcal polysaccharide antigen[105]. The arthritis often settles over the following few weeks and rarely leads to permanent deformity.

26

Gonococcal arthritis

This is the commonest cause of bacterial arthritis in normal young adults. There is a spectrum of joint disease and it is unusual to have a pure form of arthritis. Patients may have a septic monoarthritis in whom only 50% have an intra-articular organism identified. Others may present with aseptic arthritis and features consistent with a HLA B27-reactive arthritis[106] and it is argued that this infection is best classified within the SARA group of arthropathies[107]. Patients can also develop a systemic disease (disseminated gonococcal infection) with skin lesions, fleeting polyarthritis without joint effusions, tenosynovitis and positive blood cultures. This latter syndrome is related to complement activation by circulating immune complexes[108] and the bacterial lipopolysaccharide[109]. The peptidoglycan fragment of the bacteria may be the important antigenic stimulant[110]. The gonococci causing DGI are complement resistant[111], a contributing factor to the varied clinical manifestations that can occur with this organism[112].

Intestinal bypass arthritis

This arthritis is iatrogenic and follows surgery for gross obesity. Arthritis occurs in 15% of patients 2–30 months after surgery[113] and is commoner after jejunocolic rather than jejunoileal anastamosis[114]. Musculoskeletal manifestations vary from a non-specific arthralgia with tenosynovitis to an inflammatory process resembling a seronegative rheumatoid arthritis. Even seropositive erosive disease has been described[115]. Involvement of the spine is rare. The polyarthritis is characterized by excessive pain and tenderness[116]. Skin lesions occur in the majority of patients and are often macular, vesicular or even vaculitic over the arms, legs, trunk and face. It is suggested that the extra-intestinal complications are related to bacterial overgrowth within a blind loop which results in formation of immune complexes and cryoprecipitates[117–120]. This is supported by improvement in both joint and skin manifestations following antibiotic treatment or bowel reanastomosis[121]. Blind loops associated with other conditions have also been implicated as causes of a similar arthritis[122]. There are reports of bowel diseases causing an equivalent clinical picture even in the

27

absence of a blind loop[123], and, recently, the same condition has been reported in cystic fibrosis[124].

HLA B27-related reactive arthritis

It is recognized that individuals with HLA B27 are susceptible to developing arthritis after certain infections[125]. Two theoretical mechanisms have been proposed. The first is molecular mimicry where there are 'B27-like' antigenic epitopes on bacteria[126]. This either results in failure by the body to recognize bacteria as foreign, allowing them to proliferate, or in production of cross reactive antibodies which cause tissue damage. In the second theory, a microbial product (?plasmid) has a special affinity for B27, so infection leads to the plasmid attaching to the histocompatibility antigen, HLA B27, on lymphocytes and, in some unspecified way, causing arthritis[127,128]. It may be a combination of both theories[129]. An increasing number of infectious triggers have been recognized[130,131], not all due to Gram-negative organisms[132,133] and some still require identification[134]. Confirmation of a precipitating infection is often lacking and diagnosis may rest on clinical features[135]. It has been suggested that all the B27-related arthropathies have common features and can be analysed from one aetiopathological standpoint[136]. The common clinical features seen in this nebulous group of arthropathies are: urethritis, diarrhoea, conjunctivitis, anterior uveitis, arthritis, oral ulceration, circinate balanitis, keratoderma blenorrhagia, dactylitis, cardiovascular manifestations, achilles tendinitis, plantar fasciitis and other enthesopathies. These and other features can be present to varying degrees and nosology should not receive undue attention. Reiter's syndrome represents a severe subset of disease within the spectrum of reactive arthritis. It is commoner in men, often between the ages of 20 and 40 years. The triggering infection is usually sexually acquired (sexually acquired reactive arthritis, SARA)[137] or enterically acquired infection (enteric acquired reactive arthritis, EARA). Similar reactive arthropathies and spondarthritis have been associated with suppurative skin diseases, i.e. acne fulminans[138], acne conglobata[139] and plantar palmar pustulosis[140]. While some patients may only have a single episode of arthritis, others have recurrent or persistent disease[141]. Patients with the features of

28

Reiter's syndrome seem more likely to develop chronic disease[142–146]. The possession of HLA B27 predisposes to chronicity and the development of features such as iritis and spinal disease. Subtypes of HLA B27 may be important[147,148] as may other genetic factors[91] but their relationship to disease severity is not clear. The *in vitro* lymphoproliferative response against the organism is high in patients with yersinia gastroenteritis but is reduced in those patients complicated by a reactive arthritis. This response to enteric bacteria is also lower in patients with spondarthritis[149]. However, the *in vitro* lymphoproliferative response of synovial lymphocytes to the precipitating organism is maintained in reactive arthritis[150]. This infers that the initial and subsequent host response are important in the development of arthritis and that the interaction between HLA B27 and organisms is important[151,152]. Although HLA B27 is not present in all cases, the 'B27-associated reactive arthritis' has been proposed and can be examined from two aetiological standpoints.

EARA (enteric acquired reactive arthritis)

'I have finally come to the conclusion
that a good reliable set of bowels is worth
more to a man than any quantity of brains'.
Josh Billings, 1865

It is perhaps this attitude that led to therapies such as colonic lavage for many ailments, including arthritis. By chance, there was a grain of truth contained in such folklore. It is now a scientifically plausible idea that certain bacteria within specific bowels are capable of inducing both acute and chronic disease, including arthritis.

EARA often occurs in the second or third week after the gastrointestinal illness, with asymmetric joint involvement and fever. The organisms associated with EARA seem to have an affinity for affecting the gut immune system. Not only do they appear to be capable of inducing arthritis but they exacerbate inflammatory bowel disease[153,154]. This increased activity is recognized as having a temporal relationship to enteropathic arthritis. Although circulating immune complexes do occur after uncomplicated gastroenteritis[155], they do

29

appear to be related to arthritis[156,157]. This suggests that an important reaction is taking place within the immune system at the bowel lumen/wall interface, resulting in an arthritogenic factor[158]. It may be the IgA response that is important[159], as has been suggested for yersinia arthritis and spondarthritis[160-162].

Shigella flexneri

Reactive arthritis was described following an epidemic of diarrhoea in Finland when 344 patients developed Reiter's syndrome 1–90 days after infection with *Shigella flexneri*[163]. A review of 100 cases 20 years later showed that 80% continued to have articular symptoms, particularly those patients with HLA B27[143]. An epidemic of dysentery on a naval vessel confirmed this relationship[164]. It is not clear if there is more than one serotype associated with arthritis[165]. Certainly *Shigella sonnei* had not been implicated[166].

Salmonella

Infection with this organism can be followed by reactive arthritis 5–14 days after diarrhoea[167,168]. This illness need not be severe and silent carriage of the organisms has been associated with arthritis[169]. Different strains appear to be capable of inducing reactive arthritis[170,171]. Unlike shigella, this organism may produce a septic arthritis or low-grade vertebral osteomyelitis, particularly in patients with sickle cell disease.

Yersinia enterocolitica

This organism can produce an acute intestinal disease which mimics Crohn's disease. Following infection, a reactive arthritis may develop[172], often in HLA B27 + ve patients[173,174]. A complex of arthritis and erythema nodosum may also occur but in genetically different individuals. Some patients develop monoarthritis, others spondarthritis; even a picture resembling rheumatoid arthritis has been reported[175]. The diagnosis of active infection is based on isolation of the organism from faeces, blood and lymph nodes or retrospectively on serology. False-positive tests to brucella and salmonella can occur with this infection[176].

Campylobacter

This organism is a common cause of acute bacterial diarrhoea complicated by reactive arthritis[177] in up to 20% of patients[178]. The organism also causes a septic arthritis[179].

Reactive arthritis following antibiotic-induced pseudomembranous colitis has been described. The relationship to HLA B27 is not established[180,181].

SARA (sexually acquired reactive arthritis)

Post-venereal reactive arthritis develops in 1–3% of patients[182] with non-gonococcal urethritis (NGU). The risk of arthritis is increased in patients with HLA B27. The obligate intracellular pathogen, *Chlamydia trachomatosis*, causes the majority of cases of NGU in men and cervicitis in women. Although the majority of sexually acquired reactive arthritis are attributed to chlamydia[183], other pathogens are probably important[82,83,107,137,184]. The organism resembles bacteria rather than a virus and is dependent on the host cell for survival. It is important to recognize that infection may be asymptomatic and all patients with an unspecified reactive arthritis should be examined to exclude the presence of a treatable urethritis/prostatitis or cervicitis. It is claimed that intra-articular 'chlamydial elementary bodies' are responsible for the arthritis[185]; however, this requires confirmation. It has been shown that treatment with antibiotics does not help the arthritis despite clearing the urogenital infection[137]. Animal studies have shown that once arthritis is established, antibiotics are not beneficial[186]. Use of a condom during sexual intercourse may protect against further urogenital infection and exacerbation of disease. Psittacosis has also been associated with a migratory polyarthritis[187] which

31

can mimic rheumatic fever[188], indicating that chlamydial infection at other sites may be important.

INFECTION AND ANIMAL MODELS OF ARTHRITIS

In animals, it is recognized that both live organisms and their debris are capable of inducing arthritis. During the acute phase of a septic arthritis, live organisms can be recovered; this is less likely when the chronic inflammatory process has become established. This relationship is recognized in both the natural and laboratory forms of bacterial-induced animal arthritis.

Mycoplasma

Pigs and rabbits infected with mycoplasma develop an acute arthritis in which the organism can be demonstrated within the joint. During later stages, the organism disappears despite a progressive arthritis. This suggests either sequestration of antigen within the joint[189] or that the inflammatory process has become self-perpetuating[190].

Erisipelothrix rhusiopathiae

This organism is a small Gram-positive non-motile coccobacillus. In man, it causes skin infection, and, in pigs, a fluctuating arthritis. The organism is isolated from arthritic pig joints during the acute phase, but, as the arthritis progresses, the majority of joints become sterile with synovial histology showing lymphocytic infiltration[191].

Adjuvant arthritis

This arthritis is induced by intradermal injection of Freund's complete adjuvant into susceptible strains of rats[192]. It is an emulsion of heat-treated acid-fast bacilli, mineral oil and emulsifying agent. After 10–14 days, arthritis and periostitis develop. Both host factors[193] and presence of other organisms[194,195] may modulate the response. Peptidoglycans within the bacterial cell walls is believed to be the arthritogenic agent[196]. Extensive extra-articular calcification and ankylosis of joints resembles a spondarthritis rather than rheumatoid arthritis[197].

Streptococcal arthritis in rats

Injection of streptococcal cell wall fragments into the peritoneum of rats induces a chronic arthritis[198]. A proliferative inflammatory erosive synovitis develops within a week and progresses to a chronic arthritis. This resembles rheumatoid arthritis more than adjuvant, and the presence of rheumatoid factors has been described[199]. A similar model has been described following intraperitoneal injection of cell wall fragments from other bacteria[200,201].

Intra-articular bacteria in rabbits

This model demonstrates how organisms have the ability to produce different patterns of joint damage. It is dependent on the initiating organism and host response. Intra-articular injection of live organisms induces an acute suppurative arthritis from which live organisms can be recovered. Following this phase, different patterns are observed. *Staphylococcus aureus* persist within the joint and continue to produce damage. Less virulent organisms are eradicated before joint damage occurs. Gram-negative organisms produce a sterile chronic synovitis with continuing joint damage[202,203]. Even intravenous injection of Gram-negative bacterial products can induce arthritis and rheumatoid factors[204].

Clostridium perfringens

A protein-enriched diet-induced arthritis in pigs is associated with an increased faecal count of *Clostridium perfringens*. This organism is reported to be increased in the faecal flora of rheumatoid patients[205].

Because rheumatoid arthritis was thought to be a disease confined

33

to human beings, this has slowed down any major advances in the understanding and therapy of this disease. It is now known that dogs develop a similar disease with nodules, radiological erosions and autoantibodies[206,207]. Although no infective cause has yet been identified, this naturally occurring animal disease would seem a potentially useful model to exploit. Primates also develop a disease similar to rheumatoid[208] but attempts to identify a transmissible organism from humans to baboons have failed[209].

SPECULATIVE CAUSES OF CHRONIC ARTHRITIS

Rheumatoid arthritis

The 'autoimmune' label attached to rheumatoid arthritis does not exclude an infective cause. Rheumatoid factor is an antibody to altered gammaglobulin and is sometimes found in normal people. It also occurs in many bacterial diseases (subacute bacterial endocarditis, tuberculosis, syphilis, leprosy). The presence of infection can not only seroconvert individuals, but also increases the titre of a rheumatoid factor[210]. Bacterial endocarditis is associated with musculoskeletal manifestations[211] and treatment with antibiotics reduces the titre of rheumatoid factor[212]. Rheumatoid factor production results from polyclonal B lymphocyte activation, which, in vitro, can be induced by a number of mitogens, e.g. Epstein Barr virus, pokeweed, bacteria[213], mycoplasmas[214] and peptidoglycans[215]. Rheumatoid factor may represent a primitive humoral response following bacterial exposure[216] by reacting directly with the organism[199]. IgM rheumatoid factor may also amplify a low-level IgG response[217] by binding to IgG-coated organisms, hence causing complement activation[218].

Rheumatoid factor production in normals is not HLA associated[219] yet, in rheumatoid arthritis, it is linked with DRW4[220] which may represent a 'soil and seed phenomenon'. It has been proposed that rheumatoid arthritis is a gut-associated arthritis[221–224]. Olhagen suggested a link with *Clostridium perfringens* in the faecal flora of rheumatoid arthritis patients[205,225] but its aetiological significance has remained unproven[226]. Evidence that suggested chronic bacterial infection within joints[227] would seem dubious[228]. Diphtheroids and bacterial L forms have been isolated from rheumatoid arthritic joints[229,230] but their role in causing rheumatoid arthritis has not been substantiated[231]. Mycoplasmas were also implicated[232] because of animal arthritis[233] and because gold salts inactivated these organisms. However, tetracycline treatment is not beneficial for rheumatoid arthritis and makes active infection unlikely[234]. Positive serology implicating an organism should be cautiously interpreted as raised titres to mycoplasma[235], *Clostridium perfringens*[225], diphtheroids[236] and *Proteus miralbis*[237] have been found in rheumatoid arthritis. The pathogenic role of these organisms in rheumatoid arthritis remains uncertain. Mycobacteria have aroused suspicion as the cause of rheumatoid[238]. These ubiquitous organisms do have profound effects on the immune system[239] and have been implicated in other granulomatous 'autoimmune' conditions[240]. Rheumatoid disease does have a disease spectrum like mycobacterial diseases[241,242]. Evidence also suggests cross reactivity between rheumatoid lymphocytes, joint cartilage and mycobacterium[243].

Ankylosing spondylitis

There are many overlapping features between reactive arthritis, Reiter's syndrome and ankylosing spondylitis. It is recognized that some patients with chronic Reiter's syndrome may develop a disease indistiguishable from ankylosing spondylitis. Therefore, it is not surprising that a causative organism for ankylosing spondylitis has been sought. *Klebsiella pneumoniae* was thought a likely candidate because it cross reacted with HLA B27-positive lymphocytes[244]. Other evidence has pointed to a causative role with increased faecal counts related to disease activity and the presence of klebsiella antibodies[245-247]. It now seems that the organism alone is not responsible. There is a factor in a klebsiella culture supernatant capable of modifying the lymphocytes. The factor appears to be a plasmid (extrachromosomal genetic material[248-250]) and can transfer to other organisms the ability to modify B27 + ve lymphocytes[251]. Evidence now suggests that other enteric organisms are capable of producing cross reactivity with HLA B27[127] and antibody production in ankylosing spondylitis[252].

DISCUSSION

The recognition of septic arthritis in a patient with chronic joint disease is a fundamental lesson in rheumatology teaching. If this complication is missed or not treated appropriately a significant morbidity and mortality results. Infection elsewhere is also a challenge when treating the chronic arthritic. Greater understanding of why arthritics are prone to infection allied to improved antibiotics and surgical techniques has improved the overall outcome. The most exciting, at times philosophical, association between infection and arthritis is that of aetiopathogenesis. It is well recognized that transient arthralgia is a common feature of many infections[253]. This is in contrast to chronic joint sepsis which is relatively rare yet important to recognize. Many of the organisms causing joint sepsis also cause a sterile reactive arthritis. There are classifications describing the relationship between infection and arthritis but they seem limited and unable to represent the broad spectrum of arthritic events that can be associated with a single organism. The phenomenon of an arthritogenic organism producing arthritis by a number of different mechanisms is dependent on the portal of infection and host response. It is essential that we learn from known relationships and question the role of infection in rheumatic diseases of unknown cause. With improving techniques and some serendipity, specific infections causing subsets of arthritis may be found. However, it seems unlikely that a single organism will be responsible for many of the commoner heterogeneous group of chronic arthropathies. There may be a common denominator; it is possible that peptidoglycans found in the outer membrane of bacteria are important[254-257]. Bacteria may cause disease by other mechanisms, such as by being host to both bacteriophages and plasmids. Plasmids replicate within the bacterial cytoplasm and encode genes responsible for transfer of DNA. Plasmids also carry genes for antibiotic resistance and can even affect plant cell replication by transfer of DNA. It is this latter ability to affect other living cells that may be important in inducing human disease. Plasmids have been implicated in the pathogenesis of ankylosing spondylitis[258] and may play an important role in other conditions.

Although the organism may be the triggering factor, present knowledge suggests that host response is equally important in the patho-

36

genesis of arthritis. In rheumatoid arthritis, investigators have claimed subgroups of patients with an acute onset of disease in whom the prognosis is good[259–261]. There are many possible reasons: perhaps this subgroup are able to mount a host response capable of eradicating the offending organism. Inflammation is related to cytokines which can directly affect infection[262,263] as well as governing the cellular response. They also induce the acute phase response, important for clearing of damaged cells and micro-organisms[264]. The HLA status, important in governing the host response, can dictate the clinical problem. For instance, infections that cause reactive arthritis in B27 + ve individuals, can produce erythema nodosum and arthritis in different genotypes[174,265,266]. Regulation of the mucosal immune response[267], particularly the role of IgA[268], requires further investigation in rheumatic diseases. The ability to prevent bacteria becoming embedded in mucosal surfaces may be important and may not be immune based. Secretion of blood group antigens inhibits bacterial adherence[269,270] and the ability of streptococci to adhere to mucosal surfaces is probably important in rheumatic fever[271]. There is preliminary evidence that ankylosing spondylitis may be associated with ABO non-secretors[272]. The broad spectrum of other host factors includes age, gender, control of arachidonic acid metabolism, acute phase response, complement, and humoral and cellular immunity. Over the next few years, further understanding of the interface between environment (?bacteria) and host will clarify the aetiopathogenesis of many more rheumatic diseases.

REFERENCES

1. Forestier, J. (1934–1935). Rheumatoid arthritis and its treatment by gold salts: the results of six years experience. *J. Lab. Clin. Med.*, **20**, 827–840
2. Marmion, B.P. and Goodburn, G. M. (1961). Effect of an organic gold salt on Eaton's primary atypical pneumonia agent and other observations. *Nature (London)*, **189**, 247–248
3. Svarz, N. (1942). Salazopyrine, a new sulfamilamide preparation. *Acta Med. Scand.*, **6**, 577–598
4. Feltelius, N. and Hallgren, R. (1986). Sulphasalazine in ankylosing spondylitis. *Ann. Rheum. Dis.*, **45**, 396–399
5. Pullar, T., Hunter, J. A. and Capell, H. A. (1983). Sulphasalazine in rheumatoid arthritis: a double blind comparison of sulphasalazine with placebo and sodium aurothiomalate. *Br. Med. J.*, **287**, 1102–1104

6. Pullar, T., Hunter, J. A. and Capell, H. A. (1985). Which component of sulphasalazine is active in rheumatoid arthritis? *Br. Med. J.*, **290**, 1535–1538
7. McConkey, B., Davies, P., Crockson, R. A., Crockson, A. P., Butler, M. and Constable, T. J. (1976). Dapsone in rheumatoid arthritis. *Rheum. Rehab.*, **15**, 230–234
8. Ash, G., Baker, R., Rajapakse, C. and Swinson, D. R. (1986). Study of sulphamethoxazole in rheumatoid arthritis. *Br. J. Rheumatol.*, **3**, 285–287
9. Brun-Buisson, C. J. L., Saada, M., Trunet, P., Rapin, M., Roujeau, J. C. and Revuz, J. (1985). Haemolytic streptococcal gangrene and non-steroidal anti-inflammatory drugs. *Br. Med. J.*, **290**, 1786
10. Cobb, S., Anderson, F. and Baurer, W. (1953). Length of life and cause of death in rheumatoid arthritis. *N. Engl. J. Med.*, **249**, 553–556
11. Baum, J. (1971). Infection in rheumatoid arthritis. *Arthritis Rheum.*, **14**, 135–137
12. Gaulhofer de Klerck, E. H. and Van Dam, G. (1963). Septic complications in rheumatoid arthritis. *Acta Rheum. Scand.*, **9**, 254–263
13. Huskisson, E. C. and Hart, F. D. (1972). Severe unusual and recurrent infections in rheumatoid arthritis. *Ann. Rheum. Dis.*, **32**, 118–121
14. Dinand, H., Hissink, J., Muller, W., van den Berg-Loonen, E. M., Nijenhuis, L. E. and Engelfriet, C. P. (1980). HLA DRW4 in Felty's syndrome. *Arthritis Rheum.*, **23**, 1336
15. Heyn, J. (1982). Non-articular Felty's syndrome. *Scand. J. Rheumatol.*, **11**, 47–48
16. Armstrong, R. D., Fernandes, L., Gibson, T. and Kauffman, E. A. (1983). Felty's syndrome presenting without arthritis. *Br. Med. J.*, **287**, 1620
17. Barnes, C. G., Turnbull, A. L. and Vernon-Roberts, B. (1971). Felty's syndrome: a clinical and pathological survey of 21 patients and their response to treatment. *Ann. Rheum. Dis.*, **30**, 359–374
18. Goldberg, J. and Pinals, R. S. (1980). Felty's syndrome. *Semin. Arthritis Rheum.*, **10**, 52–65
19. Sienknecht, C. W., Urowitz, M. B., Pruzanski, W. and Stein, H. B. (1977). Felty's syndrome. Clinical and serological analysis of 34 cases. *Ann. Rheum. Dis.*, **36**, 500–507
20. Hurd, E. R. (1978). Presence of leucocyte inclusions in spleen and bone marrow of patients with Felty's syndrome. *J. Rheumatol.*, **5**, 26–32
21. Breedveld, F. C., Lafeber, G. J. M., De Vries, E., van Krieken, J. H. J. M. and Cats, A. (1986). Immune complexes and the pathogenesis of neutropenia in Felty's syndrome. *Ann. Rheum. Dis.*, **45**, 696–702
22. Vincent, P. C., Levi, J. A. and MacQueen, A. (1974). The mechanism of neutropenia in Felty's syndrome. *Br. J. Haematol.*, **27**, 463–475
23. Rosenthal, F. D., Beeley, J. M., Gelsthorpe, K. and Doughty, R. W. (1974). White-cell antibodies and the aetiology of Felty's syndrome. *Q. J. Med.*, **43**, 187–203
24. Weisman, M. and Zvaifler, N. J. (1976). Cryoimmunoglobulinemia in Felty's syndrome. *Arthritis Rheum.*, **19**, 103–110
25. Goldberg, L. S., Bacon, P. A., Bucknall, R. C., Fitchen, J. and Cline, M. J. (1980). Inhibition of human bone marrow – granulocyte precursors by serum from patients with Felty's syndrome. *J. Rheumatol.*, **7**, 275–278
26. Joyce, R. A., Boggs, D. R., Chervenick, P. A. and Lalezari, P. (1980). Neutrophil kinetics in Felty's syndrome. *Ann. J. Med.*, **69**, 695–702

27. Abdou, N. I., Napombejara, C., Balentine, L. and Abdou, N. L. (1978). Suppressor cell mediated neutropenia in Felty's syndrome. *J. Clin. Invest.*, **61**, 738–743

28. Hurd, E. R., Andreis, M. and Ziff, M. (1977). Phagocytosis of immune complexes by polymorphonuclear leucocytes in patients with Felty's syndrome. *Clin. Exp. Immunol.*, **28**, 413–425

29. Bodel, P. T. and Hollingsworth, J. W. (1966). Comparative morphology, respiration and phagocytic function of leukocytes from blood and joint fluid in rheumatoid arthritis. *J. Clin, Invest.*, **45**, 580–589

30. Howe, G. B., Fordham, J. N., Brown, K. A. and Currey, H. L. F. (1981). Polymorphonuclear cell function in rheumatoid arthritis and in Felty's syndrome. *Ann. Rheum. Dis.*, **40**, 370–375

31. Gupta, R. C., Laforce, F. M. and Mills, D. M. (1976). Polymorphonuclear leukocyte inclusions and impaired bacterial killing in patients with Felty's syndrome. *J. Lab. Clin. Med.*, **88**, 183–193

32. Stahl, N. I., Klippel, J. H. and Decker, J. L. (1979). Fever in systemic lupus erythematosus. *Am. J. Med.*, **67**, 935–940

33. Walport, M. and Lachmann, P. (1984). C3 receptors, complement deficiency and SLE. *Br. J. Rheumatol.*, **1**, 3–5

34. Schifferli, J. A. and Peters, D. K. (1983). Complement, the immune-complex lattice, and the pathophysiology of complement-deficiency syndromes. *Lancet*, **2**, 957–959

35. Colver, G. B., Chattopadhyay, B., Francis, R. S. and Kunzlu, K. M. N. (1981). Arthritis of the subtalar joint due to mycobacterium fortuitum. *Br. Med. J.*, **2**, 469–470

36. Halsey, J. P., Reeback, J. S. and Barnes, C. G. (1982). A decade of skeletal tuberculosis. *Ann. Rheum. Dis.*, **41**, 7–10

37. Allen, S. C. (1981). A case in favour of Poncet's disease. *Br. Med. J.*, **2**, 952

38. Bloxham, C. A. and Addy, D. P. (1978). Poncet's disease: para-infective tuberculous polyarthropathy. *Br. Med. J.*, **1**, 1590

39. Ganado, W. and Craig, A. J. (1958). Brucellosis myelopathy. *J. Bone Joint Surg.*, **40**A, 1380–1388

40. Public Health Laboratory Service (1984). Brucellosis in Britain. *Br. Med. J.*, **289**, 817

41. Kelly, P. J., Martin, W. J., Schirger, A. and Weed, C. A. (1960). Brucellosis of the bones and joints experience with thirty-six patients. *J. Am. Med. Assoc.*, **174**, 347–353

42. Marshall, R. W. and Hall, A. J. (1983). Brucellar spondylitis presenting as right hypochondrial pain. *Br. Med. J.*, **2**, 550–551

43. Norton, W. L. (1984) Brucellosis and rheumatic syndromes in Saudi Arabia. *Ann. Rheum. Dis.*, **43**, 810–815

44. Joshi, D. V., Prakash, O. and Talvar, G. P. (1971). Antigenic analysis of different strains of brucella. *Indian J. Med. Res.*, **59**, 1225–1230

45. Alarcon, G. S., Bocanegra, T. S., Gotuzzo, E., Hinostroza, S., Carillo, C., Vasey, F. B., Germain, B. F. and Espinoza, L. R. (1981). Reactive arthritis associated with brucellosis: HLA studies. *J. Rheumatol.*, **8**, 621–625

46. Gotuzzo, E., Alarcon, G. S., Bocanegra, T. S., Carillo, C., Guerra, J. C., Rolands, I. and Espinoza, L. K. (1982). Articular involvement in human bru-

cellosis: A retrospective analysis of 304 cases. *Semin. Arthritis Rheum.*, **12**, 245–255

47. Dawes, P. T. and Ghosh, S. K. (1985). Tissue typing in brucellosis. *Ann. Rheum. Dis.*, **44**, 526–528
48. Hodinka, L., Gomor, B., Meretey, K., Zahumenszky, Z. Geher, P., Telegdy, L. and Bozsoky, S. (1978). HLA-B27-associated spondylarthritis in chronic brucellosis. *Lancet*, **1**, 499
49. Caughey, D. E. and Bywaters, E. G. L. (1963). The arthritis of Whipples syndrome. *Ann. Rheum. Dis.*, **22**, 327–335
50. Knox, D. L., Bayless, T. M. and Pittman, F. E. (1976). Neurological disease in patients with treated Whipple's disease. *Medicine*, **55**, 467–476
51. Kelly, J. J. and Weisiger, B. B. (1963). The arthritis of Whipple's disease. *Arthritis Rheum.*, **6**, 615–632
52. Canoso, J. J., Saini, M. and Hermos, J. A. (1978). Whipple's disease and anklyosing spondylitis: Simultaneous occurrence in HLA-B27 positive male. *J. Rheum.*, **5**, 79–84
53. Feurle, G. E. (1985). Association of Whipples disease with HLA B27. *Lancet*, **1**, 1336
54. Hawkins, C. F., Farr, M., Morris, C. J., Hoare, A. M. and Williamson, N. (1976). Detection by electron microscope of rod-shaped organisms in synovial membrane from a patient with the arthritis of Whipple's disease. *Ann. Rheum. Dis.*, **35**, 502–509
55. Dobbins, W. O. (1981). Is there an immune deficit in Whipple's disease? *Dis. Sci.*, **26**, 247–252
56. Schmid, G. P. (1985). The global distribution of Lyme disease. *Rev. Infect. Dis.*, **7**, 41–50
57. Steele, A. C., Bartenhagen, N. H., Craft, J. E., Hutchinson, G. J., Newman, J. H., Rahn, D. W., Sigal, L. H., Spieler, P. N., Stenn, K. S. and Malawista, S. E. (1983). The early clinical manifestations of Lyme disease. *Ann. Intern. Med.*, **99**, 76–82
58. Afzelius, A. (1909). Report to Verhandlungen der dermatologischen Gesellshaft za Stockholm. *Arch. Derm Syph.*, **101**, 405–406
59. Ackermann, R., Runne, U., Klenk, W. and Dienst, C. (1980). Erythema chronicum migrans with arthritis. *Dtsch. Med. Wochen.*, **105**, 1779–1781
60. Mallecourt, J. M., Landurean, M. and Wirth, A. M. (1982). Lyme disease: a clinical case observed in western France. *Nouvelle Presse Medicale*, **11**, 39
61. Williams, D., Rolles, C. J. and White, J. E. (1986) Lyme disease in a Hampshire child – medical curiosity or beginning of an epidemic. *Br. Med. J.*, **292**, 1560–1561
62. Herzer, P., Wilske, B., Preac, M. V. and Schierz, G. (1986). Lyme arthritis: Clinical features, serological and radiographic findings of cases in Germany. *Klin. Wochensch*, **64**, 206–215
63. Steere, A. C., Malawista, S. E., Snydman, D. R., Shope, R. E., Andiman, W. A. Ross, M. R. and Steele, F. M. (1977). Lyme arthritis: an epidemic of oligoarticular arthritis in children and adults in three Connecticut communities. *Arthritis Rheum.*, **20**, 7–17
64. Goldings, E. A. and Jericho, J. (1986). Lyme disease. *Clin. Rheum. Dis.*, **2**, 343–367
65. Mertz, L. E., Wobig, G. H., Duffy, J. and Katzmann, J. A. (1985). Ticks, spi-

rochetes, and new diagnostic tests for Lyme disease. *Mayo Clin. Proc*, **60**, 402–406

66. Reik, L., Smith, L., Khan, A. and Nelson, W. (1985) Demyelinating encephalopathy in Lyme disease. *Neurology*, **35**, 267–269
67. Aberer, E., Neumann, R. and Stanke, G. (1985). Is localised scleroderma a Borrelia infection? *Lancet*, **2**, 278
68. Steere, A. C., Malawista, S. E., Hardin, J. A., Ruddy, S., Askenasey, P. W. and Andiman, W. A. (1977). Erythema chronicum migrans and Lyme arthritis. The enlarging clinical spectrum. *Ann. Intern. Med.*, **86**, 685–698
69. Kristoferistsch, W., Mayr, W. R., Partsch, H., Neumann, R. and Stanek, G. (1986). HLA-DR in Lyme Borreliosis. *Lancet*, **2**, 278
70. Sigal, L. H., Steere, A. C. and Dwyer, J. M. (1984). Evolution of cellular reactivity to the Lyme spirochete: concentration of joint fluid, *Arthritis Rheum.*, **27**, S36
71. Moffat, C. M., Sigal, L. H., Steere, A. C., Freeman, D. H. and Dwyer, J. M. (1984). Cellular immune findings in Lyme disease: correlation with serum IgM and disease activity. *Am. J. Med.*, **77**, 625–632
72. Argen, R. J. and Dixon, A. St. J. (1963). Cluttons joints and keratitis and periostitis; a case reort with histology of synovium. *Arthritis Rheum.*, **6**, 341–348
73. Reginato, A. J., Schumacher, H. R., Jumenez, S. and Maurer, K. (1976). Synovitis in secondary syphilis: Clinical, light and electron microscopic studies. *Ann. Rheum*, **22**, 170–175
74. Johnson, D. W. (1950). The Australian Leptospirosis. *Med. J. Aust.*, **2**, 724–731
75. Sutliff, D. W., Shepard, R. and Dunham, W. B. (1953). Acute Leptospira pomona arthritis and myocarditis. *Ann. Intern. Med.*, **39**, 134–140
76. Jacobs, J. H. (1951). Spondylitis following Weils disease. *Ann. Rheum. Dis.*, **10**, 61–64
77. Winter, R. J. D., Richardson, A., Lehner, M. J. and Hoffbrand, B. I. (1984). Lung abscess and reactive arthritis: rare complications of leptospirosis. *Br. Med. J.*, **288**, 448–449
78. McGill, R. C., Martin, A. M. and Edmunds, P. N. (1966). Rat bite fever due to Streptobacillus moniliformis. *Br. Med. J.*, **1**, 1213–1214
79. Hernandez, L. A., Urquhart, G. E. D. and Dick, W. C. (1977). Mycoplasma pneumoniae infection and arthritis in man. *Br. Med. J.*, **2**, 14–16
80. Weinstein, M. P. and Hall, C. B. (1974). Mycoplasma pneumoniae infection associated with migratory polyarthritis. *Am. J. Dis. Child.*, **127**, 125–126
81. Ponka, A. (1979). Arthritis associated with Mycoplasma pneumoniae infection. *Scand. J. Rheumatol.*, **8**, 27–32
82. Shepard, M. C. (1970). Non-gonococcal urethritis associated with human strains of 'T' mycoplasmas. *J. Am. Med. Assoc.*, **211**, 1335–1340
83. Bowie, W. R. (1984). Nongonococcal urethritis. *Urol. Clin. Am.*, **11**, 55–64
84. Webster, A. D. B., Loewi, G., Dourmashkin, R. D., Golding, O. N., Ward, D. J. and Asherton, G. L. (1976). Polyarthritis in adults with hypogammaglobulinaemia and its rapid response to immunoglobulin treatment. *Br. Med. J.*, **1**, 1314–1316
85. So, A. K. L., Furr, P. M., Taylor-Robinson, D. and Webster, A. D. B. (1983). Arthritis caused by Mycoplasma salivarum in hypogammaglobulinaemia. *Br. Med. J.*, **1**, 762–763

86. Taylor-Robinson, D., Gumpel, J. M., Hill, A. and Swannell, A. J. (1978). Isolation of mycoplasma pneumonia from the synovial fluid of a hypogammaglobulinaemic patient in a survey of patients with inflammatory polyarthropathy. *Ann. Rheum. Dis.*, **37**, 180–182
87. Johnston, C. L. W., Webster, A. D. B., Taylor-Robinson, D., Rapaport, G. and Hughes, G. R. V. (1983). Primary late-onset hypogammaglobulinaemia associated with inflammatory polyarthritis and septic arthritis due to Mycoplasma pneumoniae. *Ann. Rheum. Dis.*, **42**, 108–110
88. Goldenberg, D. L. (1983). Postinfectious arthritis: new look at an old concept with particular attention to disseminated gonococcal infection. *Am. J. Med.*, **74**, 925–928
89. Hadler, N. M. and Granovetter, D. A. (1978). Phlogistic properties of bacterial debris. *Semin. Arthritis Rheum.*, **8**, 1–16
90. Ford, M. J., Hurst, N. P. and Nuki,, G. (1983). Reactive arthritis – infectious agents and genetic susceptibility in the pathogenesis of sero-negative arthritis. *Scott. Med. J.*, **28**, 34–41
91. Brewerton, D. A. (1984). A reappraisal of rheumatic diseases and immunogenetics. *Lancet*, **2**, 799–802
92. Zabriskie, J. B. and Freimer, E. H. (1966). An immunological relationship between the group A streptococcus and mammalian muscle. *Exp. Med.*, **124**, 661–678
93. Kaplan, M. H. (1963). Immunological relation of streptococcal and tissue antigens. I. Properties of an antigen in certain strains of group A streptococci exhibiting an immunologic cross-reaction with human heart tissue. *J. Immunol.*, **90**, 595–606
94. Kaplan, M. H. (1976). Autoimmunity in rheumatic fever. Relationship to streptococcal antigens cross reactive with valve fibroblasts, myofibres and smooth muscle. In Dumonde, D. C. (ed.) *Infection and Immunology in the Rheumatic Diseases*, pp. 113–118. (Oxford: Blackwell Scientific Publications).
95. Zabriskie, J. B. (1976). Rheumatic fever: a streptococcal-induced autoimmune disease? In Dumonde, D. C. (ed.) *Infection and Immunology in the Rheumatic Diseases*, pp. 97–111. (Oxford: Blackwell Scientific Publications)
96. Barnert, A. L., Terry, E. E. and Persellin, R. H. (1975). Acute rheumatic fever in adults. *Am. Med. Assoc.*, **232**, 925–928
97. McDanald, E. C. and Weisman, M. H. (1978). Articular manifestations of rheumatic fever in adults. *Ann. Intern. Med.*, **89**, 917–920
98. Selby, C. L. (1985). Review and differential diagnosis of Jaccoud's arthropathy. *Int. Med. Spec.*, **6**, 55–70
99. Pinals, R. S. and Ropes, M. W. (1964). Meningococcal arthritis. *Arthritis Rheum.*, **7**, 241–258
100. Whittle, H. C., Abdulla, M. T., Fakunle, F. A., Greenwood, B. M., Bryceson, A. D. M., Parry, E. M. O. and Turk, J. I. (1973). Allergic complications of miningococcal disease. I – Clinical aspects. *Br. Med. J.*, **2**, 733–737
101. Herrick, W. W. and Parkhurst, G. M. (1919). Meningococcus arthritis. *Am. J. Med. Sci.*, **158**, 745–753
102. Rosen, M. S., Myers, A. R. and Dickey, B. (1985). Meningococcaemia presenting as septic arthritis pericarditis and tenosynovitis. *Arthritis Rheum.*, **28**, 576–578
103. Kidd, B. L., Hart, H. H. and Grigor, R. R. (1985). Clinical features of meningococcal arthritis: a report of 4 cases. *Ann. Rheum. Dis.*, **44**, 790–792

104. Greenwood, B. M., Whittle, H. C. and Bryceson, A. D. M. (1973). Allergic complications of meningococcal disease. II – Immunological investigations. *Br. Med. J.*, **2**, 737–740
105. Whittle, H. C., Greenwood, B. M., Davidson, N., McTomkins, A., Tugwell, P., Warrell, D. A., Zalin, A., Bryceson, A. D. M., Parry, E. H. O., Brueton, M., Duggan, M., Oomen, J. M. V. and Rajkovic, A. D. (1975). Meningococcal antigen in diagnosis and treatment of group A meningococcal infections. *Am. J. Med.*, **58**, 823–828
106. Rosenthal, L., Olhagen, B. and Ek, S. (1980). Aseptic arthritis after gonorrhoea. *Ann. Rheum. Dis.*, **39**, 141–146
107. Olhagen, B. (1983). Urogenital syndromes and spondarthritis. *Br. J. Rheum.*, **22**, (S2) 33–40
108. Walker, C. C., Ahlia, T. D., Tung, K. S. K. and Williams, R. C. Jr. (1978). Circulating immune complexes in disseminated gonorrhoeal infection. *Ann. Intern. Med.*, **89**, 28–33
109. Scherer, R. and Braun-Falco, O. (1976). Alternative pathway complement activation: A possible mechanism inducing skin lesions in benign gonococcal sepsis. *Br. J. Dermatol.*, **95**, 303–309
110. Fleming, T. J., Wallsmith, D. E. and Rosenthal, R. S. (1986). Arthropathic properties of gonococcal peptidoglycan fragments: implications for the pathogenesis of disseminated gonococcal disease. *Infect. Immunol.*, **52**, 600–608
111. Schoolnik, G. K., Buchanan, T. M. and Holmes, K. K. (1976). Gonococci causing disseminated gonococcal infection are resistant to the bactericidal action of normal serum. *J. Clin. Invest.*, **58**, 1163–1173
112. Rice, P. A. and Goldenberg, D. C. (1981). Clinical manifestations of disseminated infection caused by Neisseria gonorrhoeae are linked to differences in bactericidal reactivity of infecting strains. *Ann. Intern. Med.*, **95**, 175–178
113. Ginsberg, J., Quismorio, F. P., DeWind, L. T. and Mongan, E. S. (1979). Musculoskeletal symptoms after jejunoileal shunt surgery for intractable obesity: Clinical and immunologic studies. *Am. J. Med.*, **67**, 443
114. Editorial (1983). Intestinal byass syndrome. *Lancet*, **2**, 1419–1420
115. Drenick, E. J., Bassett, L. W. and Storley, T. M. (1984). Rheumatoid arthritis associated with jejunoileal bypass. *Arthritis Rheum.*, **27**, 1300–1305
116. Utsinger, P. D., Farber, N., Shapiro, R. F., Ely, P. H., McLaughlin, G. E. and Wiesner, K. B. (1978). Clinical and immunological study of the post-intestinal bypass arthritis–dermatitis syndrome. *Arthritis Rheum.*, **21**, 599
117. Wands, J. R., Lamond, J. T., Mann, E. and Isselbacher, K. J. (1976). Arthritis associated with intestinal-bypass procedure for morbid obesity. *N. Engl. J. Med.*, **294**, 121–124
118. Clegg, D. O., Samuelson, C. O., Williams, H. J. and Ward, J. R. (1980). Articular complications of jejunoileal bypass surgery. *J. Rheumatol.*, **7**, 65–70
119. Utsinger, P. D. (1979). Systemic immune complex disease after bypass surgery. *Arthritis Rheum.*, **22**, 668
120. Zapanta, M., Aldo-Benson, M., Biegel, A. and Madura, J. (1979). Arthritis associated with jejunoileal bypass. *Arthritis Rheum.*, **22**, 711–717
121. Stein, H. B., Schlappner, O. L. A., Boyko, W., Gourlay, R. H. and Reeve, C. E. (1981). The intestinal bypass arthritis – dermatitis syndrome. *Arthritis Rheum.*, **24**, 684–690
122. Klinkoff, A. V., Stein, H. B. Schlappner, O. T. A. and Boyko, W. B. (1985). Post

43

gastrectomy blind loop syndrome. *Arthritis Rheum.*, **28**, 214–217
123. Jorizzo, J. L., Apisarnthanarax, P., Subrt, P., Hebert, A. A., Henry, J. C., Raimer, S. S., Dinehart, S. M. and Reinarz, J. A. (1983). Bowel bypass syndrome without bowel bypass: Bowel associated dermatosis–arthritis syndrome. *Arch. Intern. Med.*, **143**, 457–461
124. Summers, G. D. and Webley, M. (1986). Episodic arthritis in cystic fibrosis: A case report. *Br. J. Rheum.*, **4**, 393–395
125. Brewerton, D. A., Caffrey, M., Nicholls, A., Walters, D., Oates, J. K. and James, D. C. O. (1973). Reiter's disease and HL-A27. *Lancet*, **2**, 996–998
126. Ebringer, A. and Ghuloom, M. (1986). Ankylosing spondylitis, HLA B27 and Klebsiella: cross reactivity and antibody studies. *Ann. Rheum. Dis.*, **45**, 703–709
127. McGuigan, L. E., Prendergast, J. K., Geczy, A. F., Edmonds, J. P. and Bashir, H. V. (1986). Significance of non-pathogenic cross reactive bowel flora in patients with ankylosing spondylitis. *Ann. Rheum Dis.*, **45**, 566–571
128. Geczy, A. F., Alexander, K., Bashir, H. V., Edmonds, J. P., Upfold, L. and Sullivan, J. (1983). HLA-B27, Klebsiella and ankylosing spondylitis: biological and chemical studies. *Immunol. Rev.*, **70**, 23–50
129. Van Bohemen, ChG. and Zanen, H. C. (1986). Germs and joints. *Lancet*, **2**, 1400–1401
130. Ebringer, R. (1979). Spondyloarthritis and the post-infectious syndromes. *Rheum. Rehab.*, **18**, 218–226
131. Olhagen, B. (1980). Post infectious or reactive arthritis. *Scand. J. Rheumatol.*, **9**, 193–202
132. Valtonen, V. V., Leirisalo, M., Pentikainen, P. J., Rasenen, T., Seppala, I., Larinkari, U., Ranki, M., Koskinies, S., Malkariaki, M. and Makela, P. H. (1985). Triggering infections in reactive arthritis. *Ann. Rheum. Dis*, **44**, 399–405
133. Hughes, B. R. and Hind, C. R. K. (1983). Reactive arthritis associated with staphylococcus epidermis peritonitis in a patient underlying continuous ambulatory peritoneal dialysis. *Br. Med. J.*, **286**, 188–189
134. Richens, J. E., Prasad, M. L., Bhatia, K. and Tung, M. (1986). Arthritis and HLA-B27 in Papua New Guinea. *Br. Med. J.*, **2**, 1209
135. Lionarons, R. J., Zoereh, M. V., Verhogen, J. N. and Lamers, H. A. (1986). HLA B27 associated reactive spondylarthropathy. *Ann. Rheum. Dis.*, **145**, 141–143
136. Editorial (1986). Bowel flora and ankylosing spondylitis. *Lancet*, **2**, 1259
137. Keat, A. C., Maini, R. N., Nkwarzi, G. C., Pegrum, G. D., Ridgway, G. L. and Scott, J. T. (1978). Role of chlamydia trachomatis and HLA B27 in sexually acquired reactive arthritis. *Br. Med. J.*, **1**, 605–607
138. Durter, L. L. and Hensinger, R. N. (1980). Destructive arthritis associated with acne fulmious: a rare case report. *Ann. Rheum. Dis.*, **39**, 403–405
139. Rosner, I. A., Richter, D. E., Huethner, T. L., Kuffner, C. H., Wisnieski, J. J. and Burg, C. G. (1982). Spondylarthropathy associated with hidradenitis supportiva and acne conglobata. *Ann. Intern. Med.*, **97**, 520–525
140. Sonozaki, H., Misui, H., Miyanaga, Y., Okitsu, K., Igarashi, M., Hayashi, Y., Matsuura, M., Azuma, A., Okai, K. and Kawashima, M. (1981). Clinical features of 53 cases with pustulotic arthro-oestitis. *Ann. Rheum. Dis.*, **40**, 547–553
141. Csonka, G. W. (1972). Reiter's disease. *Br. J. Hosp. Med.*, **7**, 8–12
142. Fox, R., Calin, A., Gerber, R. C. and Gibson, D. (1979). The chronicity of

symptoms and disability in Reiter's syndrome: An analysis of 131 consecutive patients. *Ann. Intern. Med.*, **91**, 190–193

143. Sairanen, E., Paronen, I. and Mahonen, H. (1969). Reiter's syndrome: A follow up study. *Acta Med. Scand.*, **185**, 57–63

144. Weinberger, H. W., Ropes, M. W., Kulka, J. P. and Bauer, W. (1962). Reiter's syndrome, clinical and pathological observations: a long term study of 16 cases. *Medicine*, **41**, 35–91

145. Good, A. E. (1962). Involvement of the back in Reiter's syndrome: follow-up study of thirty-four cases. *Ann. Intern. Med.*, **57**, 44–59

146. Calin, A. and Fries, J. F. (1976). An 'experimental' epidemic of Reiter's syndrome revisited. Follow up evidence on genetic and environmental factors. *Ann. Intern. Med.*, **84**, 564–566

147. Sikora, K., Webster, S., Sachs, J. and Festenstein, H. (1978). Associated clinical syndromes in a patient homozygous for HLAB27. *Br. Med. J.*, **1**, 1184–1185

148. Ziff, M. and Cohen, S. B. (eds.) (1985). *Advances in Inflammation Research, Vol. 9, The Spondylarthropathies*. (New York: Raven Press)

149. Sheldon, P. J. and Pell, P. A. (1985). Lymphocytic proliferative response to bacterial antigens in B27-associated arthropathies. *Br. J. Rheumatol.*, **24**, 11–18

150. Ford, D. K., da Roza, D. M. and Schulzer, M. (1985). Lymphocytes from the site of disease but not blood lymphocytes indicate the cause of arthritis. *Ann. Rheum. Dis.*, **44**, 701–710

151. Weisenhutter, C. W., Brenner, M. B., Kobayashi, S., Huberman, A. and Yu, D. T. Y. (1982). Participation of HLA molecules in the interaction between human lymphocytes and a Reiter's disease-causing bacterium. *Arthritis Rheum.*, **24**, S38

152. Brenner, M. B., Kobayashi, S., Weisenhutter, C. W., Hubberman, A. K., Bales, P. and Yu, D. T. Y. (1984). In vitro T lymphocyte proliferative response to Yersinia enterocolitica in Reiter's syndrome. *Arthritis Rheum.*, **27**, 250–257

153. Newman, A. and Lambert, J. R. (1980). Compylobacter jejuni causing flare up in inflammatory bowel disease. *Lancet*, **2**, 919

154. LaMont, J. T. and Trnka, Y. (1980). Therapeutic implications of Clostridium dofficile toxin during relapse of chronic inflammatory bowel disease. *Lancet*, **1**, 381–383

155. Briem, H., Norberg, R., Johnsson, M., *et al.* (1980). Circulating immune complexes in patients with intestinal infections. *J. Infect.*, **2**, 215–220

156. Manicourt, D. H. and Orloff, S. (1981). Immune complexes in polyarthritis after salmonella gastroenteritis. *J. Rheumatol.*, **8**, 613–620

157. Leirisalo, M., Gripenberg, M., Julkunen, I., and Repo, H. (1984). Circulating immune complexes in yersinia infection. *J. Rheumatol.*, **11**, 365–368

158. Mielants, H. and Veys, E. M. (1984). Inflammation of the ileum in patients with B27-positive reactive arthritis. *Lancet*, **1**, 288

159. van Bohemen, Ch. G., Nabbe, A. J. J. M. and Zanen, H. C. (1985) IgA response during accidental infection with Shigella flexneri. *Lancet*, **2**, 673

160. Granfors, K. and Toivanen, A. (1986). IgA anti yersinia antibodies in yersinia triggered reactive arthritis. *Ann. Rheum. Dis.*, **45**, 561–565

161. Calguneri, M., Swinburne, L., Shinebaum, R., Cooke, E. M. and Wright, V. (1981). Secretory IgA: immune defence pattern in ankylosing spondylitis and klebsiella. *Ann. Rheum. Dis.*, **40**, 600–604

162. Cowling, P., Ebringer, R. and Ebringer, A. (1980). Association of inflammation

with raised serum IgA in ankylosing spondylitis. *Ann. Rheum. Dis.*, **39**, 545–549
163. Paronen, I. (1984). Reiter's disease; a study of 344 cases observed in Finland. *Acta Med. Scand. (Suppl. 212)*, **131**, 1984
164. Noer, H. R. (1966). An 'experimental' epidemic of Reiter's syndrome. *J. Am. Med. Assoc.*, **198**, 693–698
165. Simon, D. G., Kaslow, R. A., Rosenbaum, J., Kaye, R. L. and Calin, A. (1981). Reiter's syndrome following epidemic shigellasis. *J. Rheumatol*, **8**, 969–971
166. Kaslow, R. A., Ryder, R. W. and Calin, A. (1979). Search for Reiter's syndrome after an outbreak of Shigella sonnei dysentery. *J. Rheumatol.*, **6**, 562–566
167. Vartiainen, J. and Hurri, L. (1964). Arthritis due to Salmonella typhimurium. Report of twelve cases of migratory arthritis in association with salmonella typhimurium infection. *Acta Med. Scand.*, **175**, 771–776
168. Jones, R. A. K. (1977). Reiter's disease after Salmonella typhimurium enteritis. *Br. Med. J.*, **1**, 1391
169. Trull, A. K., Eastmond, C. J., Panayi, G. S. and Reid, T. M. S. (1986). Salmonella reactive arthritis: serum and secretory antibodies in eight patients identified after a large outbreak. *Br. J. Rheumatol.*, **25**, 13–19
170. Stein, H. B., Abdulla, A., Robinson, H. S. and Ford, D. K. (1980). Salmonella reactive arthritis in British Columbia. *Arthritis Rheum.*, **23** (2), 206–210
171. Jones, R. A. K. (1977). Reiter's disease after Salmonella typhimurium enteritis. *Br. Med. J.*, **1**, 1391
172. Ahvonen, P., Sievers, K. and Aho, K. (1969). Arthritis associated with Yersinia enterocolitica infection. *Acta Rheum. Scand.*, **15**, 232–253
173. Aho, K., Ahvonen, P., Lassus, A., Steyers, K., and Tiilikainen, A. (1974). HL-A27 in reactive arthritis. A study of Yersinia arthritis and Reiter's disease. *Arthritis Rheum.*, **17**, 521–526
174. Leirisalo, M., Skylv, G., Kousa, M., Voipio-Pulkki, L. M., Suoranta, H., Nissila, M., Hvidman, L., Nielsen, E. D., Svejgaard, A., Tilikainen, A. and Laitineno, O. (1982). Follow up study on patients with Reiter's disease and reactive arthritis, with special reference to HLA-B27. *Arthritis Rheum.*, **25**, 249–259
175. Granfors, K., Isomaki, H., von Essen, R., Maatela, J., Kalliomaki, J. L. and Tiovanen, A. (1983). Yersinia antibodies in inflammatory joint disease. *Clin. Exp. Rheumatol.*, **1**, 215–218
176. Ahvonen, P. (1972). Human Yersinosis in Finland *Ann. Clin. Res.*, **4**, 30–38
177. Berden, J. H. M., Muytjens, H. L. and Van de Putte, L. B. A. (1970). Reactive arthritis associated with campylobacter jejuni enteritis. *Br. Med. J.*, **1**, 380–381
178. Gumpel, J. M., Martin, C. and Sanderson, P. J. (1981). Reactive arthritis associated with campylobacter enteritis. *Ann. Rheum. Dis.*, **40**, 64–65
179. Kovalec, J. K., Kaminski, Z. C. and Kray, P. R. (1980). Campylobacter arthritis. *Arthritis Rheum.*, **23** (1), 92–94
180. Rothschild, B. M., Masi, A. T. and June, P. L. (1977). Arthritis associated with ampicillin colitis. *Arch. Intern. Med.*, **137**, 1605–1607
181. Bolton, R. P., Wood, G. M. and Losowski, M. S. (1981). Acute arthritis associated with clostridium difficile colitis. *Br. Med. J.*, **283**, 1023–1024
182. Morton, R. S. (1972). Reiter's disease. *Practitioner*, **209**, 631–638
183. Editorial (1985) Is Reiter's syndrome caused by Chlamydia? *Lancet*, **1**, 317–319
184. Szanto, E. and Hagenfeldt, K. (1979). Sacroiliitis and salpingitis. *Scand. J. Rheumatol.*, **8**, 129–135
185. Keat, A., Thomas, B., Dixey, J., Osborn, M., Sonnex, C. and Taylor-Robinson,

D. (1987). Chlamydia trachomatis and reactive arthritis: the missing link. *Lancet*, **1**, 72–74

186. Gilbert, R. J., Schachter, J., Engleman, E. P. and Meyer, K. F. (1973). Antibiotic therapy in experimental bedsonial arthritis. *Arthritis Rheum.*, **16**, 30–33
187. Schaffner, W., Drutz, D. J., Duncan, G. W. and Koenig, M. G. (1967). The clinical spectrum of endemic psittacosis. *Arch. Intern. Med.*, **119**, 433–443
188. Simpson, R. W., Huang, C. and Grahame-Smith, D. G. (1978). Psittacosis masquerading as rheumatic fever. *Br. Med. J.*, **1**, 694–695
189. Washburn, L. R., Cole, B. C. and Ward, J. R. (1982). Chronic arthritis of rabbits induced by mycoplasmas. *Arthritis Rheum.*, **25**, 937–945
190. Washburn, L. R., Cole, B. R. and Ward, J. R. (1980). Chronic arthritis of rabbits induced by mycoplasma. *Arthritis Rheum.*, **23**, 837–845
191. Drew, R. A. (1972). Erysipelothrix arthritis in pigs as a comparative method for rheumatoid arthritis. *Proc. R. Soc. Med.*, **65**, 994–998
192. Pearson, C. M. (1956). Development of arthritis, periarthritis and periostitis in rats given adjuvant. *Proc. Soc. Exp. Biol. Med.*, **91**, 95–101
193. Battisto, J. R., Smith, R. N. Beckman, K., Sternlicht, M. and Welles, W. L. (1982). Susceptibility to adjuvant arthritis in DA and F344 rats. *Arthritis Rheum.*, **25**, 1194–1200
194. Kohashi, O., Kohashi, Y., Takahashi, T., Ozawa, A. and Shigematsu, N. (1986). Suppressive effect of E-coli on adjuvant-induced arthritis in germ free rats. *Arthritis Rheum.*, **29**, 547–553
195. Tauneg, J. D., Leany, S. L., Cremer, M. A., Mahowald, M. L., Sandberg, G. P. and Manning, P. J. (1984). Infection with mycoplasma pulmonis modulates adjuvant and collagen induced arthritis in Lewis rats. *Arthritis Rheum.*, **27**, 943–946
196. Kohashi, O., Pearson, C. M., Watanabe, Y., Kotani, S. and Koga, T. (1976). Structural requirements for arthritogenicity of peptidoglycans from Staphylococcus aureus and Lactobacillus plantarum and analogous synthetic compounds. *J. Immunol.*, **116**, 1635–1639
197. Pearson, C. M. and Chang, Y. H. (1979). Adjuvant disease: pathology and immune reactivity. *Ann. Rheum. Dis.*, **38**, 102–110
198. Cromartie, W. J., Craddock, J. G., Schwab, J. H., Anderle, S. K. and Yang, C. H. (1977). Arthritis in rats after systemic injection of streptococcal cells or cell walls. *J. Exp, Med,*, **146**, 1585–1602
199. Bokisch, V. A., Chiao, J. W., Bernstein, D. and Krause, R. M. (1973). Homogeneous rabbit 7S anti-IgG with antibody specificity for peptidoglycan. *J. Exp. Med.*, **138**, 1184–1193
200. Lehman, T. J. A., Allen, J. B., Plotz, P. H. and Wilder, R. L. (1983). Polyarthritis in rats following the systemic injection of lactobacillus Cesei cell walls in aqueous suspension. *Arthritis Rheum.*, **26**, 1259–1265
201. Esser, R. E., Stimpson, S. A., Cromartie, W. J. and Schwab, J. H. (1985). Reactivation of streptococcal cell wall induced arthritis by homologous and heterologous cell wall polymers. *Arthritis Rheum.*, **28**, 1402–1411
202. Schurman, D. J., Mirra, J. and Ding, A. (1977). Experimental E coli arthritis in the rabbit. A model of infectious and post-infectious inflammatory synovitis. *J. Rheumatol.*, **4**, 118–128
203. Hendrix, R. W. and Fisher, M. R. (1986). Imaging of septic arthritis. *Clin. Rheum. Dis.*, **2**, 459–487

47

204. Hanglow, A. C., Welsh, C. J. R., Conn, P., Pitts, J. M., Rampling, A. and Coombs, R. R. A. (1986). Experimental induction of rheumatoid factor and joint lesions after intravenous injections of killed bacteria. *Ann. Rheum. Dis.*, **45**, 50–59
205. Olhagen, B. (1975). On the aetiopathogenesis of rheumatoid arthritis. *Ann. Clin. Res.*, **7**, 119–128
206. Heuser, W. (1980). Canine rheumatoid arthritis. *Can. Vet. J.*, **21**, 314–316
207. Bennett, D. (1986). Polyarthritis in household pets. *Rheum. Pract.*, **4**, 6–13
208. Bywaters, E. G. L. (1981). Observations on chronic polyarthritis in monkeys. *J. R. Soc. Med.*, **74**, 794–799
209. MacKay, J. M. K., Simm, A. K., McCormack, J. N., Marmion, B. P., McCraw, A. P., Duthie, J. J. R. and Gardener, D. L. (1983). Aetiology of rheumatoid arthritis: an attempt to transmit an infective agent from patients with RA to baboons. *Ann. rheum. Dis.*, **2**, 443–447
210. Waller, M., Duma, R. J., Farley, E. D. and Atkinson, J. (1971). The influence of infection on titres of antiglobulin antibodies. *Clin. Exp. Immunol.*, **8**, 451–459
211. Meyers, O. L. and Commerford, P. J. (1977). Musculoskeletal manifestations of bacterial endocarditis. *Ann. Rheum. Dis.*, **36**, 517–519
212. Carson, D. A., Bayer, A. S., Eisenberg, R. A., Lawrance, S. and Theofilopoulos, A. (1978). IgG rheumatoid factor in subacute bacterial endocarditis: Relationship to IgM rheumatoid factor and circulating immune complexes. *Clin. Exp. Immunol.*, **31**, 100–103
213. Banck, G. and Forsgren, A. (1978). Many bacterial species are mitogenic for human blood B lymphocytes. *Scand. J. Immunol.*, **8**, 347–354
214. Biberfield, G. (1977). Activation of human lymphocyte subpopulations by Mycoplasma pneumoniae. *Scand. J. Immunol.*, **6**, 1145–1150
215. Levy, R. J., Haider, M., Park, H., Tar, L. and Levinson, A. I. (1986). Bacterial peptidoglycan induces in vitro rheumatoid factor production by lymphocytes of healthy subjects. *Clin. Exp. Immunol.*, **64**, 311–317
216. Clagett, J. A. and Engel, D. (1978). Polyclonal activation: a form of primitive immunity and its possible role in pathogenesis of inflammatory diseases. *Dev. Comp. Immunol.*, **2**, 235–241
217. Clarkson, A. B. and Mellow, G. H. (1981). Rheumatoid factor-like immunoglobulin M protects previously uninfected rat pups and dams from Trypanosoma lewisi. *Science*, **214**, 186–188
218. Sabharwal, U. K., Vaughn, J. H., Fong, S., Bennett, B. H., Carson, D. A. and Curd, J. G. (1982). Activation of the classical pathway of complement by rheumatoid factors assessment by radioimmune assay for C4. *Arthritis Rheum.*, **25**, 161–167
219. Engleman, E. G., Sponzilli, E. E., Batey, M. E., Ramcharan, S. and McDevitt, H. O. (1978). Mixed lymphocyte reaction in healthy women with rheumatoid factor. Lack of association with HLA DW4. *Arthritis Rheum.*, **21**, 690–693
220. Dobloug, J. H., Forre, O., Kass, E. and Thorsby, E. (1980). HLA antigens and rheumatoid arthritis. Association between HLA-Drw4 positivity and IgM rheumatoid factor production. *Arthritis Rheum.*, **23**, 309–313
221. Bennett, J. C. (1978). The infectious etiology of rheumatoid arthritis. *Arthritis Rheum.*, **21**, 531–538
222. Editorial (1979). Rheumatoid arthritis and the gut. *Br. Med. J.*, **1**, 1104

223. Zaphiropoulos, G. C. (1986). Rheumatoid arthritis and the gut. *Br. J. Rheumatol.*, **25**, 138–139
224. Segal, A. W., Isenberg, D. A., Hajirousou, V., Tolfree, S., Clark, J. and Snaith, M. L. (1986). Preliminary evidence for gut involvement in the pathogenesis of rheumatoid arthritis. *Br. J. Rheumatol.*, **25**, 162–166
225. Mansson, I. and Olhagen, B. (1966). Intestinal clostridium perfringens in rheumatoid arthritis and other connective tissue disorders. *Acta Rheum. Scand.*, **12**, 167–174
226. Struthers, G. R. (1986). Clostridium perfrigens and rheumatoid arthritis. *Br. J. Rheum.*, **14**, 419–420
227. Bartholomew, L. E. and Bartholomew, F. N. (1979). Antigenic bacterial polysaccharide in rheumatoid synovial effusions. *Arthritis Rheum.*, **22**, 969–977
228. Pritchard, D. G., Settine, R. L. and Bennett, J. C. (1980). Sensitive mass spectrometric procedure for the detection of bacterial cell wall components in rheumatoid joints. *Arthritis Rheum.*, **23**, 608–610
229. Stewart, S. M., Alexander, W. R. M. and Duthie, J. J. R. (1969). Isolation of diphtheroid bacilli from synovial membrane and fluid in rheumatoid arthritis. *Ann. Rheum. Dis.*, **28**, 477–487
230. Pease, P. (1969). Bacterial L-forms in the blood and joint fluids of arthritic subjects. *Ann. Rheum. Dis.*, **28**, 270–274
231. Middleton, P. J. and Highton, T. C. (1975). Failure to show mycoplasms in cytopathogenic virus in rheumatoid arthritis. *Ann. Rheum. Dis.*, **34**, 369–372
232. Jansson, E., Makisara, P. and Tuuri, S. (1975). Mycoplasma antibodies in rheumatoid arthritis. *Scand. J. Rheumatol.*, **4**, 165–168
233. Taylor-Robinson, D. and Taylor, G. (1976). Do mycoplasmas cause rheumatic disease? In Dumonde, D. C. (ed.) *Infection and Immunology in the Rheumatic Diseases*, pp. 177–186 (Oxford: Blackwell Scientific Publications)
234. Skinner, M., Cathcart, E. S., Mills, J. A. and Pirials, R. S. (1971). Tetracycline in the treatment of rheumatoid arthritis: a double blind controlled study. *Arthritis Rheum.*, **14**, 727–732
235. Windsor, G. D., Nicholls, A., Maini, R. N., Edward, D. G., Lemcke, R. and Dumonde, D. C. (1974). Search for mycoplasma in synovial fluids from patients with rheumatoid arthritis; *Ann. Rheum. Dis.*, **33**, 70–74
236. Duthie, J. J. R., Stewart, S. M. and McBride, W. H. (1976). Do diphtheroids cause rheumatoid arthritis In Dumonde, D. C. (ed.) *Infection and Immunology in the Rheumatic Diseases*, pp. 171–175. (Oxford: Blackwell Scientific Publications)
237. Ebringer, A., Ptaszynska, T., Corbett, M., Wilson, C., Macafee, Y., Avakian, H., Baron, P. and James, D. C. O. (1985). Antibodies to proteus in rheumatoid arthritis. *Lancet*, **2**, 305–307
238. Editorial (1986). Rheumatoid arthritis and tuberculosis. *Lancet*, **2**, 321–322
239. Editorial (1984). Immune reactions in tuberculosis. *Lancet*, **2**, 204
240. Chiodini, R. S., Van Kruiningen, H. J., Thayer, W. R., Merkal, R. S. and Contin, J. A. (1984). The possible role of mycobacterium in inflammatory bowel disease. II An unclassified Mycobacterium species isolated from patients with Crohn's disease. *Dig. Dis. Sci.*, **29**, 1073–1079
241. Panayi, G. S. (1982). Does rheumatoid arthritis have a clinicopathological spectrum similar to that of leprosy? *Ann. Rheum. Dis.*, **41**, 102–103
242. Editorial (1982). Lepromatous rheumatoid. *Lancet*, **2**, 748–749
243. Holoshitz, J., Klajman, A., Drucker, I., Lapidot, Z., Yaretzky, A., Frenkel, A.,

49

van Eden, W. and Cohen, I. R. (1986). T lymphocytes of rheumatoid arthritis patients show augmented reactivity to a fraction of mycobacteria cross-reactive with cartilage. *Lancet*, **2**, 305–309

244. Seager, K., Bashir, H. V., Geczy, A. F., Edmonds, J. and De vere-Tyndall, A. (1979). Evidence for a specific B27-associated cell surface marker on lymphocytes of patients with ankylosing spondylitis. *Nature (London)*, **277**, 68–70

245. Ebringer, A., Baines, M. and Ptasznska, T. (1985). Spondyloarthritis, uveitis, HLA B27 and Klebsiella *Immunol. Rev.*, **86**, 101–106

246. Cowling, P., Ebringer, R, Cawdwell, D., Ishii, M. and Ebringer, A. (1977). C-reactive protein, ESR and Klebsiella in ankylosing spondylitis. *Ann. Rheum. Dis.*, **39**, 45–49

247. Eastmond, C. J., Willshaw, H. E., Burgess, S. E. P., Shinebaum, R., Cooke, E. M. and Wright, V. (1980). Frequency of faecal Klebsiella aerogenes in patients with ankylosing spondylitis and controls with respect to individual features of disease. *Ann. Rheum. Dis.*, **39**, 118–123

248. McGuigan, L. E., Geczy, A. F. and Edmonds, J. P. (1985). The immunopathology of ankylosing spondylitis – a review. *Semin. Arthritis Rheum.*, **15**, 81–105

249. Van Rood, J. J., Van Leeuwen, A. and Ivanyi, P. (1985). Blind confirmation of Geczy factor in ankylosing spondylitis. *Lancet*, **2**, 943–944

250. Geczy, A. F., Alexander, K., Bashir, H. V. and Edmonds, J. (1980). A factor(s) in Klebsiella culture filtrates specifically modifies an HLA-B27 associated cell surface component. *Nature (London)*, **283**, 782–784

251. Cameron, F. H., Russel, P. J., Sullivan, J. and Geczy, A. F. (1983). Is a Klebsiella plasmid involved in the aetiology of ankylosing spondylitis in HLA-B27 positive individuals? *Mol. Immunol.*, **20**, 563–566

252. van Bohemen, C. G., Nabbe, A. J. J. M., Goei The, H. S., Dekker-Sayes, A. J. and Zanen, H. C. (1986). Antibodies to Enterobacteriaceae in ankylosing spondylitis. *Scand. J. Rheumatol.*, **15**, 143–147

253. Dudley Hart, F. (1970). Arthralgia. *Ann. Phys. Med.*, **6**, 257–261

254. Heymer, B., Schleifer, K. H., Read, S., Zabriskie, J. B. and Krause, R. M. (1976). Detection of antibodies to bacterial cell wall peptidoglycan in human sera. *J. Immunol.*, **117**, 23–26

255. Braun, D. G. and Holm, S. E. (1970). Streptococcal anti-group A precipitans in sera from patients with rheumatic arthritis and acute glomerulonephritis. *Int. Arch. Allergy*, **37**, 216–224

256. Hadler, N. M. (1967). A pathogenic model for erosive synovitis. *Arthritis Rheum.*, **19**, 256–265

257. Park, H., Schumacher, H. R., Zeiger, A. R. and Rosenbaum, J. T. (1984). Antibodies to peptidoglycan in patients with spondyloarthritis: a clue to disease aetiology. *Ann. Rheum. Dis.*, **43**, 725–728

258. Cameron, F. H., Russell, P. J., Sullivan, J. and Geczy, A. F. (1983). Is a Klebsiella plasmid involved in the aetiology of ankylosing spondylitis in HLA B27 positive individuals? *Mol. Immunol.*, **20**, 565–566

259. Short, C. L. (1964). Long remissions in rheumatoid arthritis. *Medicine*, **43**, 401–406

260. Duthie, J. J. R., Brown, P. E, Truelove, L. H., Baragar, F. D. and Lawrie, A. J. (1964). Course and progress in rheumatoid arthritis. A further report. *Ann. Rheum. Dis.*, **23**, 193–202

261. Corrigan, A. B., Robinson, R. G., Terenty, T. R., Dick-Smith, J. B. and Walters, O. (1974). Benign rheumatoid arthritis of the aged. *Br. Med. J.*, **1**, 444–446
262. Editorial (1985). Interleukin 1 in deference of the host. *Lancet*, **2**, 536–537
263. Scuderi, P., Sterling, K. E., Lam, K. S., Finley, P. R., Ryan, K. J., Ray, C. G., Patersen, E., Slymen, D. J. and Salmon, S. E. (1986). Raised serum levels of tumour necrosis factor in parasitic infections. *Lancet*, **2**, 1364–1365
264. Pepys, M. B. (1981). C-reactive protein fifty years on. *Lancet*, **1**, 653–657
265. Lambert, M., Marion, E., Coche, E. and Butzler, J. P. (1982), Campylobacter enteritis and erythema nodosum. *Lancet*, **1**, 1409
266. Neithercut, W. D., Hudson, M. A. and Smith, C. C. (1984). Can erythema nodosum and reactive arthritis be a sequel to Shigella flexneri gastroenteritis? *Scott. Med. J.*, **29**, 197–199
267. Strober, W., Richman, L. K. and Elson, C. O. (1981). The regulation of gastrointestinal immune responses. *Immunol. Today.*, **2**, 156–161
268. Stanworth, D. R. (1985). IgA dysfunction in rheumatoid arthritis. *Immunol. Today*, **2**, 43–45
269. Blackwell, C. C., Jonsdottir, K., Hanson, M. F. and Weir, D. M. (1986). Non-secretion of ABO blood group antigens predisposing to infection by Haemophilus influenzae. *Lancet*, **2**, 687
270. Aho, K. (1980). Immunogenetics of rheumatic diseases. *Scand. J. Rheumatol.*, **38** (Suppl.), 17–23
271. Editorial (1985). Decline in rheumatic fever. *Lancet*, **2**, 647–648
272. Schinebaum, R., Blackwell, C. C., Forster, P. J. G., Hurst, N. P., Weir, D. M. and Nuki, G. (1985). Non secretion of ABO blood group antigens: a host susceptibility factor in the spondyloarthropathies. Presented at the *Eular Symposium Rome, 1986, 1GP1*, 41.

3

VIRAL INFECTIONS AND CHRONIC ARTHRITIS

A. D. WOOLF

INTRODUCTION

The cause of a variety of chronic diseases, including arthritis, has been attributed to infection almost since the discovery of bacteria. Epidemiological, genetic, laboratory and experimental observations suggest that chronic arthritis may be a sequela of infection. With the failure to identify bacteria from within joints in rheumatoid arthritis, and with the development of techniques to detect viruses, there has been recent emphasis on seeking a virus as the cause of the characteristic persistent immune response that is seen in the synovium. It was first clearly documented[1] that a virus can be associated with arthritis during an epidemic of rubella at the end of World War I. Viruses can also cause chronic inflammatory disease[2,3], can evade detection and new human viruses are now often being identified[4].

Despite 40 years of research and improving techniques, there is still no firm evidence to support such a role for viruses in the aetiology of rheumatoid arthritis[5]. It is, however, clear that some viruses, such as rubella[6] and human parvovirus B19[7,8] may cause a persistent, although non-destructive, arthropathy. Does the lack of evidence exclude a role for a viral aetiology to rheumatoid disease or other chronic arthritides? In this chapter, the difficulties of establishing a relationship between a viral infection and chronic disease; the interaction between host and virus that could lead to chronic arthritis; and the known examples of persistent arthritis cause by viruses will be discussed.

IDENTIFYING VIRUSES AS A CAUSE OF CHRONIC ARTHRITIS

There are several approaches to demonstrating a relationship between an infectious agent and disease but there are difficulties in proving this to be causal.

Determining the long-term natural history of acute viral arthritis will show whether it results in a chronic destructive arthritis but large controlled studies are required to prove such an outcome rather than the various case reports in the literature[9,10]. The epidemiological pattern of disease such as the geographic or seasonal distribution, may suggest an infectious aetiology. It was the geographic clustering without temporal relation and a peak incidence in warm weather which suggested an arthropod vector in Lyme disease[11,12].

Seroepidemiology is of limited value. It is unhelpful if the cause is a common virus and outcome is host dependent, or if a novel agent is being sought for which the appropriate serological tests will not exist. In acute infections, the timing of antibody response and of symptoms will, however, strongly suggest an association which can be shown to be causal if the study is appropriately controlled.

Electron microscopic identification of viral-like particles in synovial tissue is suggestive but the isolation of infectious virus or the identification of viral nucleic acid sequences from within the diseased joint provides the most valuable evidence for an aetiological role. Cloning techniques are becoming increasingly powerful tools to identify viral genome[13]. Isolation of virus, however, does not prove causation as it may be a mere passenger in one of the cell populations attracted to the inflammatory synovium. Rubella has been isolated from peripheral blood lymphocytes two years after vaccination[14]. In addition, the normal human genome is known to contain viral nucleic acid sequences[15,16]. It is also possible that the putative infection is a transient event or is distant from the joint, and then one would not expect to isolate it from the joint itself in established cases.

Less direct methods have been used. The demonstration of an antibody response within the joint may reflect the presence of antigen in the joint, but could also be due to polyclonal activation of B cells or result from the random trapping of plasmablasts in the joint[17]. Rheumatoid synovium is an immunologically active tissue. It makes substantial amounts of specific antibody following influenza vac-

54

cination[18], which illustrates that it can participate in a systemic immune response.

The proliferative responses of synovial lymphocytes obtained from various chronic arthropathies to antigens derived from infectious agents has been used to implicate these agents in pathogenesis[19,20]. T cells may, however, be sensitized to microbial antigens distant from the joint and non-specifically home in to the inflamed joint[21]. Although this indirect evidence of the causative antigen may give us clues, there are shortcomings that limit the conclusions that can be made[22,23].

The identification of viral products, enzymes such as reverse transcriptase of retroviruses, is another indirect means of demonstrating viral infection. Interferon production or the presence of an enzyme induced by interferon, such as 2-5A synthetase, may indicate viral infection but is non-specific[24].

Experimental models, although useful, are limited by the species specificity of viruses and differences in clinical manifestations of the same virus in different animals[25]. They may, however, provide a means of showing the putative agent to induce the disease and provide analogous models to human disease that allow detailed dissection of the interaction between virus and host and of the resultant disease process. Rabbits develop a chronic erosive arthritis following a single intra-articular injection of herpes simplex virus into the knee joint[26]. The goat retrovirus, caprine arthritis-encephalitis virus (CAEV), produces a chronic destructive arthritis which is being increasingly studied[27].

To prove a causal relationship between a virus infection and chronic arthritis is difficult[2]. Ideally the Henle–Koch postulates[28] should be fulfilled. These state that:

(1) The infectious agent occurs in every case of the disease in question and under circumstances which can account for the pathological changes and clinical course of the disease,
(2) The agent does not occur in other disease by chance, and
(3) after the agent is isolated from the body and repeatedly grown in culture, it can induce the disease anew.

The chronic diseases that are known to be caused by infectious agents, such as rheumatic fever, subacute sclerosing panencephalitis and Reiter's syndrome, do not behave as classic infections, but represent unusual responses of the host to a common, often transient, infective agent. Clearly, these would not fulfil the Henle–Koch postulates and new criteria for causation have been formulated by Evans[28] to allow for these difficulties.

In diseases recently identified as viral in origin, such as the acquired immunodeficiency syndrome (AIDS), isolating the organism has required advanced techniques which have not been applied to their full in rheumatic diseases. New viruses have often been identified following the development of new cell culture techniques – EBV with B-lymphoid cell cultures[29], HIV with T cell cultures[30] and, most recently, a new lymphotropic herpes virus (HBLV) with the activation of B cells at the start of culture[31]. The negative findings so far in chronic arthritis in no way exclude the role of viruses in its aetiology, but just disappoint and discourage researchers.

VIRUS–HOST INTERACTIONS

Most viral illnesses are acute and transient, with clearance of the virus by the immune system and life-long immunity. Many viral infections are subclinical, some recurrent and others are persistent. The outcome depends on the interaction between virus, host and the immune system (Figure 3.1).

Viruses are obligate intracellular parasites. The virus must penetrate the host and enter the cell for it to replicate and spread. Viral infection is usually cytopathic and the disease is a consequence of the number and functions of those cells affected. The selective tropism of a virus to cells may relate either to cell-surface host receptors or to cell-specific regulatory elements inside the cell. EB virus infects human B cells because they bear virus receptors which are closely associated with, but not identical to, C3 receptors[32]. The selective tropism of some retroviruses appears to be determined by viral sequences that exert transcriptional control in selected cells[33].

Viral replication is associated with the production of viral proteins and formation of virions. Organelle and cell membranes may be disrupted. Viral proteins that are inserted into the plasma membrane can provoke an immune response which is regulated by host genes

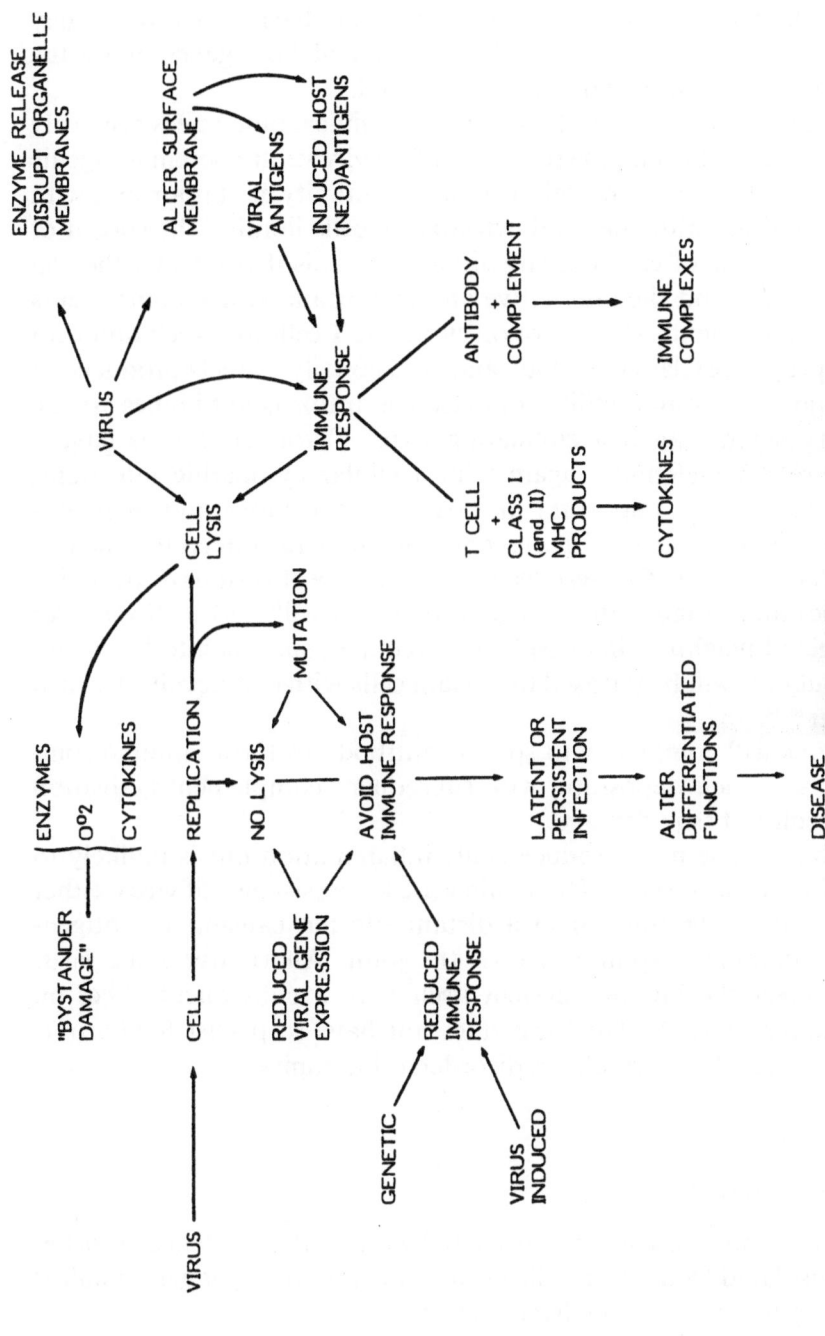

FIGURE 3.1 Viral injury to host

within the major histocompatibility complex. Host neoantigens may be induced in the cell by the derepression of host genes or by the combination of virus and host cell material.

The susceptibility to viral infection and clinical outcome is primarily determined by the immune response. Most viruses are potent antigenic stimulants. Humoral and cell-mediated immunity are important, with both antiviral antibodies and cytotoxic T cells limiting the spread of infection. Lysis of cells bearing viral antigens is dependent either on antiviral IgG and the alternative and membrane attack components of the complement pathway, or on cytotoxic T cells in association with the appropriate Class I product, and occasionally Class II products, of the major histocompatibility complex. Neutralizing antibodies are the primary defence against circulating virus. Cytotoxic T cells have a major role in defending against intracellular cytopathic infections, although they are important in most viral infections and their dys-function is associated with susceptibility to viral infections such as varicella and CMV. Cell lysis leads to the release of various degradative enzymes and inflammatory mediators which will lead to 'bystander damage' of neighbouring tissues. Cytokinines, such as interferon and interleukin I, will be released by certain cells with distinct effects, such as fever[24,34].

Virions will combine with specific antibody to form immune complexes, and their deposition with subsequent complement activation may result in tissue damage.

Such a course may produce acute inflammation but is unlikely to result in chronic disease. This could arise by persistence of virus, either locally within the joint or at a distant site but causing an antigen-specific immune response against the joint. Alternatively the virus could infect the immune system itself with a subsequent effect on immunoregulation[35]. The virus does not have to persist for chronic disease to result if it results in disordered immunity.

Viral persistence

Several chronic diseases are associated with viral persistence. Measles can be isolated from brain cells in subacute sclerosing panencephalitis and hepatitis B in chronic liver disease[36].

For a virus to persist, it must not lytically infect cells and it must avoid the host immune system. This may be either by reduced viral gene expression or by an abnormal host immune response, genetically predetermined or a direct effect of the virus on the immune system itself. A latent infection is established if the cell does not allow normal viral replication and there are detectable viral nucleic acids in the absence of infectious virus. Productive replication may be activated at some later time. A persistent infection will occur if viral replication does not result in cell lysis, and both viral nucleic acid and infectious virus are detectable.

The natural virus may have low gene expression or this may arise *de novo* by mutation during viral replication within the host (Figure 3.1). Lytic viral replication will be prevented or there may be a reduction in the expression of virally encoded surface antigens with subsequent reduction in the immune response. Latency or persistence will result. Alternatively, mutant strains may no longer interact with neutralizing antibodies or sensitized T lymphocytes and the immune response to the original strain will act as a selective force for the emergence of the novel strain. Equine infectious anaemia virus is a highly mutatable retrovirus which persists by this process[37]. In some instances, the host cell does not permit normal viral replication, which is dependent either on the cell type or on its state of differentiation. Cytomegalovirus will infect but not replicate in teratocarcinoma cells unless they are differentiated[38]. Caprine arthritis–encephalitis virus infects monocytes but this is only productive when the cells differentiate and mature into macrophages[39].

The host immune response may be avoided or impaired by the direct infection of immune cells[35] or by a genetic host abnormality. Many persistent viruses infect lymphocytes (EBV, HIV) or cells of the mononuclear phagocytic system (CAEV). They replicate, persist and spread within them. Viruses can alter specialized cell functions without affecting their vital functions[40]. Measles, influenza and cytomegaloviruses infect human peripheral blood lymphocytes *in vitro* and alter some of their specific immune functions, such as immunoglobulin production or the generation of cytotoxic cells, and HIV affects the immune response *in vivo*[41]. Lymphotropic strains could arise by mutation in the host during infection. This direct infection of the immune system will not only enable persistence of the virus, but also

59

result in other diseases related to an abnormal immune response. Tuberculosis can be reactivated by an acute measles infection, and allergy to tuberculin begins during the prodromal stage and persists for up to 6 weeks[42]. AIDS is characterized by opportunistic infections.

Susceptibility to viral diseases can be determined genetically[43]. In mice, genes have been identified that can specifically modulate the outcome of various DNA and RNA virus infections, and single genes appear to influence resistance to only a particular family or even just one species of virus. The familial occurrence of persistent viral diseases may, however, relate more to their transmission from parent to child, either vertically within the genome, in colostrum or just by close contact. No clear associations between the MHC and persistent infections have been demonstrated.

The viral genome must somehow be preserved within the cell for any long-term infection. It may become integrated into host chromosomes where it may remain silent, protected from degradation and enabled to segregate to daughter cells during host cell division (vertical transmission). Human immunodeficiency virus (HIV) is known to integrate[44], although the latent papovaviruses do not[45].

VIRAL PATHOGENESIS OF CHRONIC ARTHRITIS

A virus could cause synovitis, either by directly infecting the joint or by causing an immune response directed against the joint (Figure 3.2).

Direct infection of the synovium may result in acute inflammation by the mechanisms already discussed.

Infection outside the joint could result in antibodies to viral or virus-induced neoantigens which cross-react with synovial antigens. Antigens unique to the synovial endothelium have been identified[46]. Circulating immune complexes may be formed and deposited in the synovium. Antiidiotype antibodies that react to viral receptors on cells may form and result in disease[47]. Infection of the immune system itself could result in disordered immunoregulation with loss of suppression or non-specific stimulation of the immune response[35].

Persistence of the virus, by mechanisms as described, or the persistence of the abnormal immune response would lead to chronic arthritis. It is possible that the putative virus is not unique but rep-

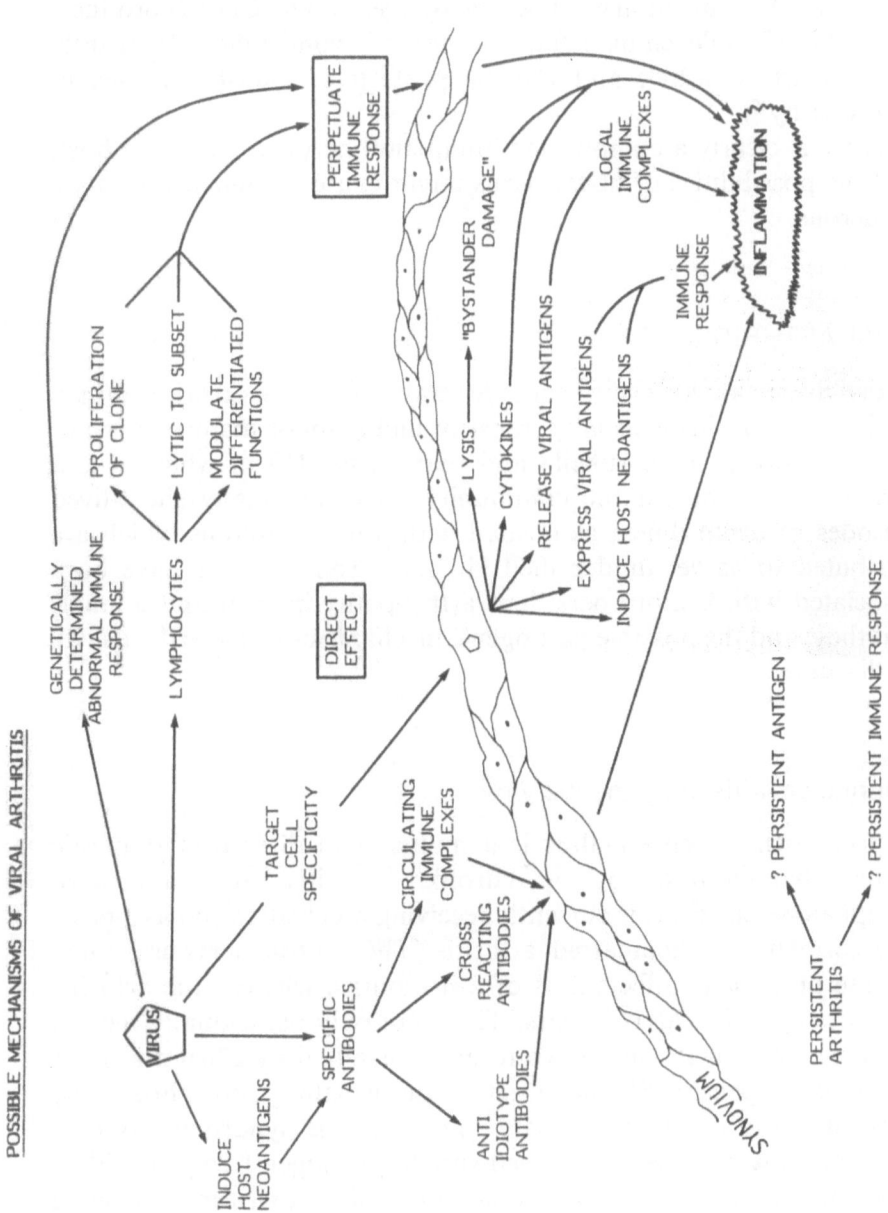

FIGURE 3.2   Possible mechanisms of viral arthrits

resents an abnormal host response to a common agent, presumably determined by genetic factors. For example, the outcome of human parvovirus B19 infection is influenced by age, sex and Class II products of the MHC: children have few symptoms[48]; women more frequently develop arthropathy[8]; and DRI is protective against a persistent arthropathy[49].

There is clearly a complicated interaction between virus and host, and the possibilities of how a virus might cause chronic arthritis are numerous.

VIRAL ARTHRITIS

Many viruses are known to cause arthralgia or frank arthritis in man (Table 3.1) but this is usually transient and a minor manifestation of infection, except with rubella and parvovirus B19 in which it is a common outcome. In the community, there are many short-lived episodes of acute illness associated with joint symptoms which are attributed to as yet unidentified viruses[50]. Some viruses have been associated with a more persistent arthropathy in man and animals and these and the possible pathogenic mechanisms of the arthritis will be discussed.

Caprine arthritis encephalitic virus

Caprine arthritis–encephalitis is a multisystem disease of domestic goats characterized by a chronic arthritis and a leuko-encephalomyelitis[27]. It is currently receiving much attention as a possible correlate to rheumatoid arthritis. The central nervous system disease principally affects kids of 2–4 months, whereas the arthritis becomes apparent at 1–2 years. These are only occasionally seen in the same animal. It was shown to be transmitted by 220 nm filtrates of tissue suspensions[51] and a retrovirus isolated from chronically affected joints of arthritic goats will cause the syndrome after its inoculation into caesarian-derived specific-pathogen-free goat kids[52]. It is a lentivirus: a non-oncogenic subfamily of retroviruses, associated with viral persistence and chronic disease[53], which include the visna-

62

TABLE 3.1   Arthritogenic viruses

Type of virus	Incidence of arthropathy in adults
DNA viruses	
Parvovirus B19	60% women 30% men
Hepatitis B	25%
Variola	Rare
Vaccinia	Rare
EBV	Rare
Cytomegalovirus	Rare
Herpes simplex	Rare
Adenovirus 7	Rare
RNA viruses	
Rubella	20–30% women 5–10% men
Rubella vaccine	20–40% women
Mumps	0.5%
ECHO	Rare
Ross River virus	Common
Chikungunya	Common
O'nyong nyong	Common

maedi virus and the equine infectious anaemia virus.

CAEV is a common infection with the prevalence of antibody ranging from 58–100% in herds in different states of the USA[54]. Most goats would appear to have a subclinical infection. Transmission is usually vertical from mother to kid by ingestion of colostrum and milk, the virus being carried within macrophages in the milk[55]. There is no evidence of vertical transmission within the germline, although integration of viral genome within the host has been described[56]. Less than 25% develop a chronic arthritis[55] which is associated with viral persistence within the joint[27].

The onset of arthritis is usually insidious, with the development of joint pain and swelling and of weight loss. The severity of arthritis fluctuates and migrates, most commonly affecting the carpal joints but also the hocks and stifle joints[55]. Some cases progress to marked loss of joint movement and deviation of the distal ends of forelimbs.

63

Other systemic features include arteritis, pericarditis, pleurisy, interstitial nephritis and amyloidosis[57]. They occasionally also have neurological involvement.

A mild synovial hyperplasia and perivascular mononuclear cell infiltrate are the earliest changes in experimentally infected goat kids[58]. The proliferation and necrosis of synovial lining cells continues, progressing to a marked synovial hyperplasia and villous hypertrophy with lymphoid follicle formation in the synovial membrane. Ia-positive cells are seen surrounded by lymphocytes which are producing α- and β-interferon[59]. Chronically arthritic goats often show large areas of cellular necrosis and necrobiosis of collagen in villi, and fibrinous concretions in synovial spaces[55,58]. Mineralization is frequently found in areas of necrosis and this is seen radiologically initially in the periarticular tissue and later in the joint capsules, ligaments, tendons and tendon sheaths. There is a minor periosteal reaction with periarticular osteophyte formation which proceeds to a roughening of the bony surfaces extending away from the joint. The cartilage surfaces are often eroded or ulcerated, resulting in irregular articular surfaces. In severe cases, subchondral bone collapses and the joint fuses[55].

Synovial fluid from an acutely inflamed joint has a low viscosity and contains 1000–20 000 cells/mm^3, 90% of which are mononuclear cells. These are predominantly lymphocytes but also synovial cells and large foamy macrophages, often containing eosinophilic clumps in their cytoplasm[55]. Rheumatoid factor is not found[27].

CAEV replicates within the joint following the innoculation of goat kids after which viral titres fluctuate widely, but can be detected at one year post infection. When undetectable in synovial fluid, the presence of CAEV has been demonstrated by co-cultivating synovial fluid cells with susceptible cells[60]. CAEV appears to persist in the joint with a low but variable level of expression for several years. Cells of the mononuclear phagocytic system, particularly macrophages, appear to be the primary cells that support CAEV replication[61].

Central questions are how does this virus persist despite a host immune response and how does it produce tissue damage? Neither can be fully answered. The infection of the mononuclear phagocytic system is a feature of several persistent viruses[35,62]. Only a minor fraction of monocytes appear to be infected with CAEV *in vivo*, and productive infection only occurs after the cells differentiate and mature[39]. The immunologically silent nature of the infection, due to this low level of viral replication and expression, is a possible explanation for persistence, with insufficient production of viral antigens for the detection and destruction of the infected cell by the immune system. How this variable expression is controlled is unclear. The degree of integration of viral DNA may also be important in establishing persistence. CAEV fails to induce neutralizing antibodies[63], possibly due either to lack of appropriate antigenic epitopes or to an abnormal host immune response which may be constitutively deficient or impaired by the infection itself[63,64].

There are some data suggesting mechanisms of synovitis. Non-neutralizing antibodies are produced to viral surface glycoproteins and are found in the synovial fluid several years after infection. There is predominantly a polyclonal increase in IgG_1 produced locally within the joint[64], and the synovial fluid antibodies are principally directed against a 90 000 MW surface glycoprotein[65]. T-lymphocytes reactive with CAEV are found during the first 8 months but their presence becomes variable after 2–5 years[66,67]. The synovitis, measured by joint swelling, correlates with the expression of CAEV within the joint[60]. Apart from this direct interaction between CAEV and the immune system, there is a more generalized augmentation of lymphocyte reactivity, for example T-lymphocytes from infected goats show an increased proliferation *in vitro* to co-conavalin A^{27}. It has been suggested that the pathogenesis is similar to antigen-induced arthritis[27]. An initial infection initiates an immune response, but, due to its failure to clear the virus, the persistent viral antigens within the joint interact with the specifically sensitized lymhocytes to cause inflammation which may be enhanced by the non-specific augmentation of their reactivity.

It is an interesting model in which trigger and outcome are known but the mechanisms are not well understood. Of particular interest is the variable host response to a virus. It may have lessons for understanding rheumatoid disease. There is, at present, no evidence for CAEV as a cause of rheumatoid using techniques such as DNA hybridization, but even these techniques are limited, despite their sensitivity, if as few cells are infected as in the diseased goat itself.

Rubella

Rubella is a togavirus: small icosahedral enveloped single-stranded RNA viruses.

Infection with rubella is frequently subclinical or associated with a mild illness, characterized by fever, rash and lymphadenopathy, but infection during pregnancy can result in congenital abnormalities which has lead to vaccination programmes in many countries. This has altered the epidemiology of the disease.

Before the introduction of routine vaccination, epidemics occurred at 6–9-year intervals. Children of 5–9 years were most commonly affected and 80–90% of young adults had antibodies. In the USA, where immunization is directed at young children to reduce chance exposure of susceptible pregnant women, cases are now predominantly seen in older school children and young adults who have a higher incidence of constitutional symptoms and athropathy. The overall incidence of the disease is also falling from a peak of 1.8 million cases in the USA during the epidemic of 1964 to 11 795 in 1979[68] and rubella arthropathy from natural infection is now less common. Cases are seen, however, following the vaccination of seronegative young females.

Children who are symptomatic usually have a mild illness with a fine pink maculapapular rash developing on the face 14–21 days after exposure and spreading to trunk and limbs, often coalescing to give a diffuse erythema similar to scarlet fever. They may have fever, sore throat and lymphadenopathy but these prodromal symptoms are more common and severe in adults who also may have myalgia and, more specifically, eye pain. Joint symptoms are most often seen in adult women who account for up to 90% of cases. In one study, 52.2% of adult women with symptomatic rubella had frank arthritis compared with 8.7% of adult men who more often just had arthralgia[6]. Other studies would suggest a lower incidence of 20–30% of adults with clinical rubella developing joint symptoms[1,69–71] but a female predominance is clear. It is unknown how often arthropathy might be the only manifestation of rubella infection.

Frequently, there is pain and morning stiffness in the absence of objective synovitis. The onset is usually rapid with a symmetrical distribution. The small joints of the hands, knees and wrists are

66

generally affected but ankles, shoulders, elbows and hips may be involved. The course may be migratory and additive. Periarthritis, tenosynovitis and carpal tunnel syndrome occasionally occur. The arthropathy develops from one week before to one week after the rash. It usually improves within a few weeks but symptoms often persist many months, one study finding a third of those with arthritis still had symptoms at 18 months[6].

An arthropathy may also occur following vaccination with various live strains of virus[72–80]. Three strains have been developed: the HPV-77 duck embryo strain, the Cendehill strain and the RA 27/3 strain which is grown in human cell culture and is now the most widely used. The quality and quantity of antibody following RA 27/3 vaccination more closely approximates natural infection. All strains may cause myalgia, arthralgia and arthritis although the latter is less common with RA 27/3[73–81]. Children, as with the wild infection, seldom develop these systemic features, 1–10% having joint symptoms which are usually a transient mild arthralgia[73,81,82]. Joint symptoms, however, occur in up to 40% of adult women, with frank arthritis in 2–13.6% following RA 27/3[6,77,80]. There are few data on men. Severity is similar between the different strains. The arthropathy occurs usually 2–4 weeks after vaccination, either just preceding or coincident with isolation of virus from the pharynx or seroconversion. Although it generally lasts for less than 2 weeks, more persistent and often recurrent joint symptoms have been reported to last for more than 18 months[6] and some children have been symptomatic at five years following HPV-77 DK12 vaccination[83]. It is usually more persistent in those with more severe initial symptoms[6].

The pattern of arthropathy is similar to that following wild infection, but, in a direct comparison, the arthropathy following RA 27/3 was of lower incidence, less severity and shorter duration[6].

The high incidence of arthropathy and occasional isolation of rubella in wild[84] and post-vaccination[75,85] arthropathy from joints and from peripheral blood mononuclear cells[14] has lead to the suggestion that the arthropathy results from local, occasionally persistent, infection, recurrent antigenaemia and circulating immune complex (CIC) formation and deposition. This is supported by: the non-cytopathic infection of synovial cells *in vitro* with long-term production of viral antigen[86]; the finding of raised CIC levels by Clq binding[87]; and finding of CIC-containing rubella-specific IgG in adults who developed joint symptoms after immunization[88]. These complexes are not, however, specific. Rubella-specific CIC were also found in 60% of vaccinated adults without joint symptoms[89] and there is little difference between those with and without arthropathy by Clq ELISA and Raji ELISA following vaccination or wild infection as CICs were detected in some cases irrespective of symptoms[89]. This does not exclude local formation and deposition of complexes within the joint. No HLA association has been shown with the development of arthropathy[90]. The role of rubella in chronic arthritis is discussed on page 74.

Human parvovirus B19

Parvoviruses are unique in being the only single-stranded DNA viruses of vertebrates. They are the small (parvo = small) icosahedral non-enveloped particles, 18–26 nm in diameter, with a genome of only about 5.5 kb. A pathogenic human parvovirus, B19, was not identified until 1975[91], and then its disease associates were unclear. It is a common infection, with specific IgG antibodies detectable in about 60% of adults[92]. Screening sera of children for B19 fortuitously found antigen in the serum of children with homozygous sickle cell anaemia admitted with aplastic crises[93], and it has since been confirmed as a major cause of aplastic crises in various chronic haemolytic anaemias[94,95]. It will lytically infect erythroid progenitor cells in culture[96]. The autonomous parvoviruses, to which B19 appears to belong, are dependent on a host cell function transiently expressed during the S phase of the growth cycle for their own replication because of their limited genetic capacity[97]. This leads to their pathogenicity for proliferating cells, and animal parvoviruses often cause pancytopaenia and gastroenteritis. Erythema infectiosum was identified as the more usual manifestation of B19 infection in 1983[98]. This exanthematous illness was first described by Tschamer in 1889 but, because of its frequent similarity to rubella, it is often unrecognized as a distinct entity and many are unaware of its existence. Children develop a rash which is variable but often includes malar erythema ('slapped cheek'). The rash is curious in its frequent recrudescence which may occur over several months[48]. It is provoked by heat, emotion or pressure. Children have mild constitutional symptoms, affecting about 20%, which include malaise, fever, headache and 5% complain of joint pain but less than half of these note swelling[48]. Occasionally, it is severe enough to appear similar to systemic juvenile chronic arthritis but it is more transient. Adults more frequently have joint symptoms with the rash, with pain in about 75% and swelling in 60%[48]. In 1985, cases of acute arthritis associated with serological evidence of recent B19 infection, but in the absence of the typical rash, were described[7,99]. A controlled epidemiological study of the adults associated with an outbreak in a primary school has now confirmed that B19 can cause an acute, occasionally persistent, arthropathy in adults, often in the absence of the classic features of erythema infectiosum[8]. Cases were identified independent of symptoms or severity and it was found that infection can be asymptomatic in 25%. There is some concern about infection *in utero* as several cases of hydrops foetalis have been reported[100].

The arthropathy developed[101] 18 days after experimental intranasal innoculation of volunteers with B19. It is usually an acute onset symmetrical polyarthropathy with pain, most often affecting hands, feet and knees with swelling of the proximal interphalangeal joints [7,8,99]. Morning stiffness is often pronounced. The median duration of these joint symptoms is 10 days[8] but they may persist for much longer[7,8] and joint swelling, particularly of the small joints of the hands, has been noted at 21 months with arthralgias persisting longer[102]. The pattern of the arthropathy is occasionally palindromic, persisting for 5 years in one case[102], or recurrences of more widespread symptoms similar to the onset have been seen 1 year after the onset[102]. These generally last a few days and, although there is usually just arthralgia, joint swelling does occasionally occur. The arthropathy is more common and more marked in women, occurring in 60% compared with 30% of men[8]. Persistent and recurrent cases are nearly all women[7,8,99,10].

Human parvovirus B19 can clearly cause an occasionally persistent arthropathy, and, with the decline in rubella, it may be one of the commonest viral triggers, but what are the mechanisms? Age and sex clearly affect the expression of B19 infection, as is noted with other viruses, such as rubella. Less than 5% of children[8,48] but 60% of women develop joint symptoms[8].

HLA typing has shown DR1 to be absent in 32 adults with arthro-

69

pathy persisting more than 2 months, compared with 20.1% in a local control population (A. D. Woolf, personal communication) which raises the possibility that it is a marker for, or directly involved in, a more effective virus–host interaction. The prevalence of DR4 in these adults was 50%, compared with 36.2% in local controls, and this was not significant.

Virus has not been found in synovium, synovial fluid, bone marrow or peripheral blood mononuclear cells in patients with persistent arthropathy (A. D. Woolf and J. P. Clewley, personal communication) using dot hybridization with a virtually entire genome clone[103], and the specific IgM response does not persist, both arguing against viral persistence. Although immune complexes containing virus are transiently detected during the acute infection[101], this is several days before the development of rash and arthropathy, and only low levels have occasionally been found in some patients with arthropathy[7].

Rheumatoid factor has occasionally been found[7,99,104], and, although this is often in patients with only a transient arthropathy, cases have been reported where the onset of classical seropositive rheumatoid arthritis appears to be coincident with serological evidence of recent B19 infection[10]. Seroepidemiological studies have shown no difference between the incidence of past B19 infection in patients with rheumatoid arthritis and that in age- and sex-matched controls[105] (A. D. Woolf, personal communication). B19 may be acting as a trigger in certain genetically susceptible individuals[106] and some of these cases have had a haplotype which has been associated with rheumatoid arthritis[10]; or, alternatively, these cases may have been the mere coincidence of two diseases. A long-term follow-up study of B19 infection is currently trying to establish the final outcome of infection.

Hepatitis B virus

Hepatitis B virus is a small spherical DNA virus. The virion is the 42 nm Dane particle which consists of a nucleocapsid enclosed by a coat, the surface antigen (HBsAg). The core antigen (HBcAg), the e antigen (HBeAg), the partially double-stranded DNA and a DNA polymerase form the nucleocapsid.

Most people develop a transient, often subclinical, infection which is associated with an antibody response to HBsAg. If symptomatic, prodromal symptoms of fever, anorexia, nausea, vomiting and occasionally diarrhoea are followed by jaundice. There may also be a rash, either maculopapular, petechial or urticarial. About 25% of those icteric develop joint symptoms[107] but these also occur in the absence of jaundice[107,108]. The arthropathy is of interest because of the proposed pathogenic mechanisms. About 5–10% of infected people fail to clear the virus and a third of these develop chronic active hepatitis. Others develop chronic persistent hepatitis or remain asymptomatic carriers. Polyarteritis nodosa and mixed essential cryoglobulinaemia have also been associated with the hepatitis B infection[107,109].

The arthropathy usually develops during the prodromal phase but may be simultaneous with or occur after the onset of jaundice[107]. There is usually a rapid onset of joint pain and marked morning stiffness with either a migratory, additive or a symetrical pattern. Arthritis in addition to arthralgia develops[107]. Tenderness may suggest more of a periarthritis and the swelling is not always clearly synovial[110]. The small joints of the hands and knees are most often involved but also wrists, ankles, shoulders, elbows, hips and occasionally the spine[107]. Symptoms usually persist for 1–3 weeks, resolving in most with the onset of jaundice. Prolonged or recurrent joint symptoms may occur in those who have persistence of HB antigenaemia[110,111]. Subcutaneous nodules, histologically like rheumatoid nodules, have been noted[112]. Rash and fever often accompany the arthropathy but as many as 59% may remain anicteric[107,108], although most do have abnormal liver function tests. Rheumatoid factor is occasionally detected[107].

Arthropathy can develop at all ages but is infrequent in children. There is no marked sex association[107]. The incidence of arthropathy has been very high in some outbreaks and the possibility of arthritogenic viral strains has been suggested[110]. Joint symptoms also occur in multisystem vasculitis associated with hepatitis B antigenaemia, are more persistent and rheumatoid factor is often detected[107].

The acute arthropathy is thought to be a 'serum sickness'-like syndrome[113]. It occurs early in the infection and is frequently accompanied by skin involvement. There is antigenaemia with free HBsAg found in serum and synovial fluid. Anti-HBsAg antibodies are not usually found simultaneous with antigen[107] but appear as

71

HBsAg disappears, often coinciding with resolution of the arthropathy[110,114]. Complement levels are depressed in serum and synovial fluid[107,110,111,115]. Cryoglobulins containing HBsAg, anti-HBs antibody and complement components are found. These differ from those in patients without arthropathy, both quantitatively and qualitatively[115]. One difference is their ability to activate the classical and alternative pathways of complement *in vitro*[115].

Persistent HB virus antigenaemia is associated with polyarteritis nodosa (PAN)[107] and mixed essential cryoglobulinaemia (MEC)[109]: conditions both associated with deposition of immune complexes within which hepatitis B antigen has been demonstrated[109,115] but differing in the vessel size involved. This may relate to the characteristics of the immune complexes and depend on whether or not there is antigen excess and to the host immune response. Free HBsAG is found in PN[107], suggesting antigen excess associated with soluble complexes, whereas little or no free HBsAg is found in MEC[109].

Other viruses

Arthritis has been associated with other common acute viral infections (Table 3.1). These have been occasional case reports and the timing of the arthropathy to the clinical and serological evidence of infection is the only evidence for a causal association. Virus has not been isolated from the synovium.

Mumps

Mumps was first associated with an arthropathy in 1850 by Rillet[116] and less than 40 cases have been reported. It is a paramyxovirus: large pleomorphic enveloped single-stranded RNA viruses that include measles, and canine distemper virus. Persistent measles infection causes subacute sclerosing panencephalitis[117], and inclusions suggestive of a paramyxovirus have been reported in osteoclasts of Pagetic bone[118].

Mumps is subclinical in up to 40% of cases and its clinical manifestations relate to its tropism for glandular and nervous tissue. Parotitis is common but post-pubertal men may develop epididymo-orchitis and post-pubertal women, occasionally, oophoritis. Meningitis is occasionally apparant, predominantly in men, but a pleo-cytosis of the CSF has been noted in up to 62% of cases. Encephalitis occurs in about 1 in every 6000 cases.

An arthropathy occurs in less than 0.5% of clinical cases of mumps[119,120]. Most cases have been young men[121]. In some, there has been no parotitis and the diagnosis has been made retrospectively by serology. Symptoms usually follow the parotitis by 1–3 weeks and there is typically an acute polyarthritis which is often migratory. Large joints, such as the shoulders, hips, knees, and ankles, are commonly affected, although small joints, such as the metacarpophalangeal and proximal interphalangeal joints, may be involved. Others develop an acute monarthritis of knee, hip or ankle; or arthralgia alone. If children have joint symptoms, they are mild and limited to a few joints[122]. These joint symptoms have resolved in 45% by 2 weeks, but have persisted more than a month in 22% and occasionally up to 6 months[121]. X-rays have only shown soft-tissue swelling and there is no long-term damage. Other visceral involvement is often seen in those with arthritis. The pathogenesis of arthropathy remains unknown. Virus has never been isolated from the joint and no immune complexes were found in the only study done[123].

Epstein–Barr virus

Epstein–Barr virus infection may be accompanied by an acute symmetric polyarthritis lasting a few days but two more persistent cases have been reported[124,125], one having a persistent symmetrical rheumatoid factor negative erosive polyarthritis at 2 years. Three patients have been reported who developed a polyarthritis following an acute febrile illness with serological evidence of *Coxsackie B* infection. This progressed to an erosive polyarthritis in one case which was persistent at 3 years[9].

RHEUMATOID ARTHRITIS

Evidence for a viral aetiology to rheumatoid arthritis has been extensively sought[5]. Viruses remain popular as a potential cause for rheumatoid arthritis for reasons previously stated, but, even if a virus were identified, it would prove difficult to show conclusively that it is causative[2]. Several of the viral infections already discussed may persist for months to years, may be associated with rheumatoid factor[7,99,104,107], and there have been case reports of them progressing to an erosive arthropathy[9,124], occasionally classical rheumatoid arthritis[10]. To establish that a common infection progresses to rheumatoid arthritis in only a few cases requires properly controlled prospective follow-up studies that have not been done. The various methods discussed to identify a viral aetiology have been applied to rheumatoid arthritis over the last 40 years and have proved inconclusive or negative. With the failure to isolate a virus by culture, by inoculation of rheumatoid tissue into animals and humans and by other more conventional means, the idea that it might be a non-cytopathic latent virus became popular. Techniques sensitive enough to detect these, such as DNA hybridization, have all failed, but, as illustrated by CAEV, only a small population of cells need be infected which limits the ability of even these methods to identify the putative virus. Less direct methods, such as seeking viral nucleic acid polymerases, have also been unrewarding. There have been occasional reports of viral isolates in established chronic arthritis, in particular of rubella[126–128]. These have been in a variety of adult and childhood arthritides, rarely in seropositive rheumatoid arthritis, and could represent the virus being a mere passenger in one of the cell populations attracted to the already inflamed synovium[21], as rubella virus has been isolated from peripheral blood lymphocytes 2 years after vaccination[14]. A parvovirus RA-1 has been isolated from a rheumatoid joint by cocultivation with human foetal lung fibroblasts followed by repeated passage in new born mice[129]. RA-1 has only been obtained by serial passage through neonatal mice and it could be a rodent virus unrelated to rheumatoid disease. The direct identification of RA-1 antigen or DNA in rheumatoid synovium is required to prove any association, and, once specific antibody of sufficient activity is available, supportive seroepidemiological data could be sought.

74

Serology has, however, suggested a role for Epstein–Barr (EB) virus in rheumatoid arthritis. It is attractive as an aetiological agent as it is lymphotrophic, lymphoproliferative and a polyclonal B-cell activator. An immunoprecipitin to a nuclear antigen from EB-transformed B cells was found in sera from patients with rheumatoid arthritis and named RANA[130,131]. Anti-RANA antibodies react with the same molecular weight polypeptide as anti-EBNA-1 (an EBV nuclear antigen) antibodies[132] and they also react with a normal constituent of B-lymphocytes[133]. That anti-RANA antibodies may be both auto-antibody and an antibody to EBNA-1 is supported by the cross-reactivity of a monoclonal anti-EBNA-1 antibody with a normal cellular protein[134,135]. However, the specificity of anti-RANA antibodies to rheumatoid arthritis, when compared with normal controls and other chronic inflammatory diseases, is unclear as their prevalence and levels have varied in the different control groups studied[135]. In addition to this possible molecular mimicry, there are abnormalities in cellular immunity in rheumatoid arthritis relating to EB virus. There appears to be a decreased T-cell suppression of EBV-infected B-lymphocytes[136,137] and an increased frequency of EBV-infected cells in patients with rheumatoid arthritis[138], but, again, the specificity of these changes for rheumatoid arthritis is unclear. Although these data make an attractive hypothesis for the pathogenesis of rheumatoid disease[135], host or other environmental factors would have to play a role as EBV is such a ubiquitous infection.

Seroepidemiological studies have otherwise been unhelpful and would suggest either a host-dependent reaction of an individual to a common virus or a novel agent for which serological tests do not exist. There are few data at present on what genetic factors do affect outcome in the known viral arthritides, apart from the possible protective effect of DR1 in parvovirus B19 arthropathy[49], but an association between rheumatoid arthritis and DR4 is clearly established[139,140].

Local synthesis of antiviral antibodies[17] or the presence of viral-sensitized lymphocytes[20] have been sought and found, but, for reasons stated, these findings do not provide substantive evidence of a role for these viruses in chronic arthritis and there are other explanations for their presence[17,22,23].

There is, therefore, no proven role at present for viruses as a cause of the chronic arthritides, such as rheumatoid arthritis or juvenile chronic arthritis. This does not exclude such a trigger and it is still being sought. However, even in arthritides such as Reiter's disease, in which the infective trigger and the host susceptibility are known, there is still little understanding of the mechanisms of their interaction. The analysis of animal models, such as CAEV, may help to unravel the pathogenesis of viral-induced arthritis.

REFERENCES

1. Geiger, J. C. (1918). Epidemic of German measles in a city adjacent to an army cantonment. *J. Am. Med. Assoc.,* **70,** 1818–1820
2. Norden, C. W. and Kuller, L. H. (1984). Identifying infectious etiologies of chronic disease. *Rev. Infect. Dis.,* **6,** 200–213
3. Haywood, A. M. (1986). Patterns of persistent viral infections. *N. Engl. J. Med.,* **315,** 939–948
4. Editorial (1986). An unexpected new human virus. *Lancet,* **2,** 1430–1431
5. Editorial (1984). The viral aetiology of rheumatoid arthritis. *Lancet,* **1,** 772–774
6. Tingle, A. J., Allen, M., Petty, R. E., Kettyls, G. D., and Chantler, J. K. (1986). Rubella associated arthritis. I. Comparative study of joint manifestations associated with natural rubella infection and RA 27/3 rubella immunisation. *Ann. Rheum. Dis.,* **45,** 110–114
7. White, D. G., Woolf, A. D., Mortimer, P. P., Cohen, B. J., Blake, D. R. and Bacon, P. A. (1985). Human parvovirus arthropathy. *Lancet,* **1,** 419–421
8. Woolf, A. D., Campion, G. V., Chiswick, A., Wise, S., Cohen, B. J. and Dieppe, P. A. (1986). An epidemiological study of human parvovirus infection in adults. *Br. J. Rheum.,* **25** (Suppl. 1), 2
9. Hurst, N. P., Martynoga, A. G., Nuki, G., Sewell, J. R., Mitchell, A. and Hughes, G. R. V. (1983). Coxsackie B infection and arthritis. *Br. Med. J.,* **286,** 605
10. Cohen, B. J., Buckley, M. M., Clewley, J. P., Jones, V. E., Puttick, A. H. and Jacoby R. K. (1986). Human parvovirus infection in early rheumatoid and inflammatory arthritis. *Ann. Rheum. Dis.,* **45,** 832–838
11. Steere, A. C., Broderick, T. F. and Malawista, S. E. (1978). Erythema chronica migrans and Lyme arthritis – Epidemiological evidence of a tick vector. *Am. J. Epidemiol.,* **108,** 312–321
12. Steere, A. C. and Malawista, S. E. (1985). Lyme Disease. In Kelley, W. N., Ruddy, S., Sledge, C. B. and Harris, E. D. (eds.) *Textbook of Rheumatology,* pp. 1557–1563. (Philadelphia: W. B. Saunders)
13. Engleberg, N. C. and Eisenstein, B. I. (1984). The impact of new cloning techniques on the diagnosis and treatment of infectious diseases. *N. Engl. J. Med.,* **311,** 892–901
14. Chantler, J. K., Ford, D. K. and Tingle, A. J. (1981). Rubella-associated arthritis: rescue of rubella virus from peripheral blood lymphocytes two years post-vaccination. *Infect. Immunol.,* **32,** 1274–1280
15. Peden, K., Mounts, P. and Haywood, G. S. (1982). Homology between mammalian cell DNA sequences and human herpes virus genomes detected by a hybridisation procedure with high-complexity probe. *Cell,* **31,** 71–80

16. Callahan, R., Chiu, I-M., Wong, J. F. H., Pronick, S. R., Roe, B. A., Aaronson, S. A. and Schlom, J. (1985). A new class of endogenous human retroviral genomes. *Science*, **228**, 1208–1211
17. Mimms, C. A., Stokes, A. and Grahame, R. (1985). Synthesis of antibodies, including antiviral antibodies, in the knee joint of patients with arthritis. *Ann. Rheum. Dis.*, **44**, 734–737
18. Pelton, B. K., Havey, A. R. and Denman, A. M. (1985). The rheumatoid synovial membrane participates in systemic anti-viral immune responses. *Clin. Exp. Immunol.*, **62**, 657–661
19. Ford, D. K., da Roa, D. M. and Schulzer, M. (1985). Lymphocytes from the site of disease but not blood lymphocytes indicate the cause of arthritis. *Ann. Rheum. Dis.* **44**, 701–710
20. Ford, D. K. and da Roza, D. M. (1986). Further observations on the response of synovial lymphocytes to viral antigens in RA. *J. Rheumatol.*, **13**, 113–117
21. Asherson, G. I., Allwood, G. G. and Mayhew, B. (1973). Contact sensitivity in the mouse. XI. Movement of T blasts in the draining lymph nodes to sites of inflammation. *Immunology*, **25**, 485–494
22. Denman, A. M. (1986). Editorial. Lymphocytes – Dolphins or enlightening rheumatological investigators? *J. Rheumatol.*, **13**, 9–12
23. Philips, P. E. (1986). Editorial. Lymphocyte responses to viral antigens in rheumatoid arthritis. *J. Rheumatol.*, **13**, 6–8
24. Mimms, C. A. and White, D. O. (1984). Interferons. In *Vial Pathogenesis and Immunology* pp. 167–178. (Oxford: Blackwell Scientific Publications)
25. Rott, R., Herzog, S., Fleischer, B., Douglas, S. D. and Pearson, C. M. (1985). Detection of serum antibodies to Borna disease virus in patients with psychiatric disorders. *Science*, **228**, 775–756
26. Webb, F. W., Bluestone, R., Goldberg, L. S. *et al.* (1973). Experimental viral arthritis induced with herpes simplex. *Arthritis Rheum.*, **16**, 241–250
27. McGuire, T. C. (1984). Retrovirus-induced arthritis. In Notkins, A. L. and Oldstone, M. B. A. (eds.) *Concepts in Viral Pathogenesis*, pp. 254–259. (New York: Springer–Verlag)
28. Evans, A. S. (1976). Causation and disease: the Henle–Koch postulates revisited. *Yale J. Biol. Med.*, **49**, 175–195
29. Epstein, M. A. and Barr, Y. M. (1964). Cultivation in vitro of human-lymphoblasts from Burkitt's malignant lymphoma. *Lancet*, 1, 252–253
30. Barre-Sinoussi, F., Cherman, J. C., Fey, F., Nugeyre, M. T., Chamaret, F., Dauguet, C., Axler-Blin, C., Vezinet-Brun, F., Rouzioux, C., Rozenbaum, W. and Montagnier, L. (1983). Isolation of a T-lymphotropic retrovirus from a patient at risk for acquired immune deficiency syndrome (AIDS). *Science*, **220**, 868–871
31. Salahuddin, S. Z., Ablashi, D. V., Markham, P. C., Josephs, S. F., Sturzenegger, S., Kaplan, M., Halligan, G., Biberfeld, P., Wong-Staal, F., Kramarsky, B. *et al.* (1986). Isolation of a new virus, (HBLV), in patients with lymphoproliferative disorders. *Science*, **234**, 596–601
32. Wells, A., Koide, N. and Stein, H. (1983). The Epstein–Varr virus receptor is distinct from the C_3 receptor. *J. Gen. Virol.*, **64**, 449–453
33. Laimins, L. A., Gross, P., Pozzatti, R. and Khoury, G. (1984). Characterisation of enhancer elements in the long terminal repeat of Moloney murine sarcoma virus. *J. Virol.*, **49**, 183–189

34. Oppenheim, J. J., Kovacs, E. J., Matsushima, K. and Durum, S. K. (1986). There is more than one interleukin-1. *Immunology Today,* **7,** 45–56
35. Mimms, C. A. (1986). Interactions of viruses with the immune system. *Clin. Exp. Immunol.,* **66,** 1–16
36. Mimms, C. A. and White, D. O. (1984). Persistent infections. In *Viral Pathogenesis and Immunology*, pp. 200–253. (Oxford: Blackwell Scientific Publications)
37. Payne, S., Parekh, B., Montelaro, R. C. and Issel, C. J. (1984). Genomic alterations associated with persistent infections by equine infectious anaemia virus, a retrovirus. *J. Gen. Virol.,* **65,** 1395–1399
38. Gonezol, E., Andrews, P. W. and Plotkin, S. A. (1984). Cytomegalovirus replicates in differentiated but not in undifferentiated human embryonal carcinoma cells. *Science,* **224,** 159–161
39. Narayan, O., Kennedy-Stoskepf, S., Sheffer, D., Griffin, D. E. and Clements, J. E. (1983). Activation of caprine arthritis–encephalitis virus expression during maturation of monocytes to macrophages. *Infect. Immun.,* **41,** 67–73
40. Oldstone, M. B. A. (1984). Viruses can alter cell function without causing cell pathology: disordered function leads to imbalance of homeostasis and disease. In Notkins, A. L. and Oldstone, M. B. A. (eds.) *Concepts in Viral Pathogenesis*, pp. 269–276. (New York: Springer-Verlag)
41. Southern, P. and Oldstone, M. A. (1986). Medical consequences of persistent viral infection. *N. Engl. J. Med.,* **314,** 359–367
42. von Pirquet, C. (1908). Das Verhalten der Kutanen Tuberkulin-reaktion wahrend der Masern. *Dtsch. Med. Wochenschr.,* **34,** 1297–1300
43. Brinton, M. A. and Nathanson, N. (1981). Genetic determinants of virus susceptibility: epidemiologic implications of murine models. *Epidemiol. Rev.,* **3,** 115–139
44. Marx, J. L. (1985). More about the HTLVs and how they act. *Science,* **229,** 37–38
45. Chesters, P. M., Heritage, J. and McCance, D. J. (1983). Persistence DNA sequences of BK virus and JC virus in normal tissues and in diseased tissues. *J.*
46. Jalkanen, S., Steere, A. C., Fox, R. I., and Butcher, E. C. (1986). A distinct endothelial recognition system that controls lymphocyte traffic into inflamed synovium. *Science,* **233,** 556–558
47. Plotz, P. H. (1983). Autoantibodies are anti-idiotype antibodies to antiviral antibodies. *Lancet,* **2,** 824–826
48. Ager, E. A., Chin, T. D. Y. and Poland, J. D. (1966). Epidemic erythema infectiosum. *N. Engl. J. Med.,* **275,** 1326–1331
49. Woolf, A. D., Campion, G. V., Klouda, P., Chiswick, A., Cohen, B. J. and Dieppe, P. A. (1986). HLA and the clinical manifestations of human parvovirus infection. *Br. J. Rheum.,* **25** (Suppl. 2), 35
50. Utsinger, P. D., Strimel, W. H., Fite, F. L. and Hicks, J. T. (1982). Viruses are a common etiology of the syndrome of fever, acute short-lived polyarthritis and rash. *Arthritis Rheum.,* **25** (suppl.), abstract 334
51. Cork, L. C., Hadlow, W. J., Crawford, T. B., Gorham, J. R., and Piper, R. C. (1974). Infectious leukoencephalomyelitis of young goats. *J. Infect. Dis.,* **129,** 134–141
52. Crawford, T. B., Adams, D. S., Cheevers, W. P. and Cork, L. C. (1980). Chronic arthritis in goats caused by a retrovirus. *Science,* **207,** 997–999

53. Haase, A. T. (1986). Pathogenesis of lentivirus infections. *Nature (London)*, **322**, 130–135
54. Crawford, T. B. and Adams, D. S. (1981). Caprine arthritis–encephalitis: Clinical features and the presence of antibody in selected goat populations. *J. Am. Vet. Med. Assoc.*, **178**, 713–719
55. Adams, D. S., Klevjer-Anderson, P., Carlson, J. L., McGuire, T. C. and Gorham, J. R. (1983). Transmission and control of caprine-arthritis encephalitis virus. *Am. J. Vet. Res.*, **44**, 1670–1675
56. Yaniv, A., Dahlberg, J. E., Tronick, S. R., Chiu, I-M. and Aaronsen, S. A. (1985). Molecular cloning of integrated caprine in arthritis–encephalitis virus. *Virology*, **145**, 340–345
57. Crawford, T. B., Adams, D. S., Sande, R. D., Gorham, J. R. and Henson, J. B. (1980). The connective tissue component of the caprine arthritis–encephalitis syndrome. *Am. J. Pathol.*, **100**, 443–454
58. Adams, D. S., Crawford, T. B. and Klevjer-Andersen, P. (1980). A pathogenetic study of the early connective tissue lesions of viral caprine arthritis–encephalitis. *Am. J. Pathol.*, **99**, 257–278
59. Kennedy, P. G., Narayan, O., Ghotbi, Z., Hopkins, J., Gendelman, H. E., Clements, J. E. (1985). Persistent expression of Ia antigen and viral genome in visna-maedi virus-induced inflammatory cells. Possible role of lentivirus-induced interferon. *J. Exp. Med.*, **162**, 1970–1982
60. Klevjer-Anderson, P., Adams, D. S., Anderson, L. W., Banks, K. L. and McGuire, T. C. (1984). A sequential study of virus expression in retrovirus induced arthritis of goats. *J. Gen. Virol.*, **65**, 1519–1525
61. Klevjer-Anderson, P. and Anderson, L. W. (1982). Caprine arthritis–encephalitis virus infection of caprine monocytes. *J. Gen. Virol.*, **58**, 195–198
62. Bielefeldt Ohmann, H. and Babiuk, L. A. (1986). Viral infections in domestic animals as models for studies of viral immunology and pathogenesis. *J. Gen. Virol.*, **66**, 1–25
63. Narayan, O., Sheffer, D., Griffin, D. E., Clements, J. and Hess, J. (1984). Lack of neutralizing antibodies to caprine arthritis encephalitis lentivirus in persistently infected goats can be overcome by immunization with inactivated myobacterium tuberculosis. *J. Virol.*, **49**, 349–355
64. Johnson, C. G., Adams, D. S. and McGuire, T. C. (1983). Pronounced production of polyclonal IgG$_1$ in the synovial fluid of goats with caprine arthritis–encephalitis infection. *Infect. Immun.*, **41**, 805–815
65. Johnson, G. C., Barber, A. F., Klevjer-Anderson, P. and McGuire, T. C. (1983). Preferential immune response to virion-surface glycoproteins by caprine arthritis–encephalitis virus. *Infect. Immun.*, **41**, 657–665
66. Adams, D. S., Crawford, T. B., Banks, K. L., McGuire, T. C. and Perryman, L. E. (1980). Immune response of goats persistently infected with caprine arthritis–encephalitis virus. *Infect. Immun.*, **28**, 421–427
67. DeMartini, J. C., Banks, K. L., Greenlee, A., Adams, D. S. and McGuire, T. C. (1983). Augmented T lymphocyte responses and abnormal B lymphocyte numbers in goats chronically infected with the retrovirus causing caprine arthritis–encephalitis. *Am. J. Vet. Res.*, **44**, 2064–2069
68. Ray, C. G. (1983). Rubella. In Petersdorf, R. G., Adams, R. D., Braunwald, E., Isselbecher, K. J., Martin, J. B. and Wilson, J. D. (eds.) *Harrison's Principles of Internal Medicine*, 10th Edn., pp. 1115–1117. (New York: McGraw-Hill)

69. Hope Simpson, R. E. (1940). Rubella and polyarthritis. *Br. Med. J.,* **1,** 830
70. Louden, I. S. L. (1953). Polyarthritis in rubella. *Br. Med. J.,* **1,** 1388
71. Lewis, G. W. (1953). Polyarthritis in rubella. *Br. Med. J.,* **2,** 149–150
72. Farquhar, J. D. and Corretjer, J. E. (1969). Clinical experience with Cendehill rubella vaccine in mature women. *Am. J. Dis. Child.,* **118,** 266–268
73. Spruance, S. L. and Smith, C. B. (1971). Joint complications associated with derivatives of HPV-77 rubella vaccine. *Am. J. Dis. Child.,* **122,** 105–111
74. Thompson, G. R., Ferreyra, A. and Brackett, R. G. (1971). Acute arthritis complicating rubella vaccination. *Arthritis Rheum.,* **14,** 19–26
75. Weibel, R. E., Stokes, J. Jr., Buynak, E. B. and Hilleman, M. R. (1969). Rubella vaccination in adult females. *N. Engl. J. Med.,* **280,** 682–685
76. Weibel, R. E., Stokes, J. Jr., Buynak, E. B. and Hilleman, M. R. (1972). Influence of age on clinical responses to HPV-77 duck rubella vaccine. *J. Am. Med. Assoc.* **222,** 805–807
77. Weibel, R. E., Villarejos, V. M., Klein, E. B., Buynak, E. B., McLean, A. A. and Hilleman, M. R. (1980). Clinical and laboratory studies of live attenuated RA27/3 and HPV-77-DE rubella virus vaccines. *Proc. Soc. Exp. Biol. Med.,* **165,** 44–49
78. Polk, B. F., Modlin, J. F., White, J. A. and DeGirlami, P. C. (1982). A controlled comparison of joint reactions among women receiving one of two rubella vaccines. *Am. J. Epidemiol.,* **115,** 19–25
79. Fogel, A., Moshkowitz, A., Rannon, L. and Gerichter, Ch. B. (1971). Comparative trials of RA27/3 and Cendehill rubella vaccines in adult and adolescent females. *Am. J. Epidemiol.,* **93,** 392–398
80. Gerson, A. A., Frey, H. M., Borkowsky, W. and Steinberg, S. (1980). Live attenuated rubella virus vaccine: comparison of responses to HPV-77-DE5 and RA27/3 strains. *Am. J. Med. Sci.,* **279,** 95–97
81. Cooper, L. Z., Ziring, P. R., Weiss, H. J., Matters, B. A. and Krugman, S. (1969). Transient arthritis after rubella vaccination. *Am. J. Dis. Child.,* **118,** 218–225
82. Dudgeon, J. A., Marshall, W. C. and Peckham, C. S. (1969). Rubella vaccine trials in adults and children. *Am. J. Dis. Child.,* **118,** 237–242
83. Spruance, S. L., Metcalf, R., Smith, C. B., Griffiths, M. M. and Ward, J. R. (1977). Chronic arthropathy associated with rubella vaccination. *Arthritis Rheum.,* **20,** 741–747
84. Hildebrandt, H. M. and Massab, H. F. (1966). Rubella synovitis in a one-year old patient. *N. Engl. J. Med.,* **274,** 1428–1430
85. Ogra, P. L. and Herd, J. K. (1971). Arthritis associated with induced rubella infection. *J. Immunol.,* **107,** 810–813
86. Cunningham, A. L. and Fraser, J. R. E. (1985). Persistent rubella virus infection of human synovial cells cultured in vitro. *J. Infect. Dis.,* **151,** 638–645
87. Vergani, D., Morgan-Capner, P., Davies, E. T., Anderson, A. W., Tee, D. E. H. and Pattison, J. R. (1980). Joint symptoms, immune complexes and rubella. *Lancet,* **2,** 321–322
88. Coyle, P. K., Wolinsky, J. S., Buimovici-Klein, E., Moucha, R. and Cooper, L. Z. (1982). Rubella-specific immune complexes after congenital infection and vaccination. *Infect. Immun.,* **36,** 498–503
89. Singh, V. K., Tingle, A. J. and Schulzer, M. (1986). Rubella-associated arthritis. II. Relationship between circulating immune complex levels and joint manifestations. *Ann. Rheum. Dis.,* **45,** 115–119

90. Robitaille, A., Cockburn, C., James, D.C.O. and Ansell, B.M. (1976). HLA frequencies in less common arthropathies. *Ann. Rheum. Dis., 35*, 271–273

91. Cossart, Y.E., Field, A.M., Cant, B. and Widdows, D. (1975). Parvovirus-like particles in human sera. *Lancet, 1*, 73

92. Cohen, B.J., Mortimer, P.P. and Pereira, M.S. (1983). Diagnostic assays with monoclonal antibodies for the human serum parvovirus-like virus (SPLV). *J. Hyg. (London), 91*, 113–131

93. Anderson, M.J., Davis, L.R., Hodgson, J., Jones, S.E., Murtaza, L., Pattison, J.R., Stroud, C.E., White, J.M. *et al.* (1982). Occurrence of infection with a parvovirus-like agent in children with sickle cell anaemia during a two-year period. *J. Clin. Pathol., 35*, 744–749

94. Young, N. and Mortimer, P.P. (1984). Viruses and bone marrow failure. *Blood, 64*, 729–737

95. Saarinen, U.M., Chorba, T.L., Tattersall, P., Young, N.S., Anderson, L.J., Palmer, E. and Coccia, P.F. (1986). Human parvovirus B19–induced epidemic acute red cell aplasia in patients with hereditary haemolytic anaemia. *Blood, 67*, 1411–1417

96. Mortimer, P.P., Humphries, R.K., Moore, J.G., Purcell, R.H. and Young, N.S. (1983). A human parvovirus-like virus inhibits haematopoetic colony formation in vitro. *Nature (London), 302*, 426–429

97. Cotmore, S.F. and Tattersall, P. (1984). Characterisation and molecular cloning of a human parvovirus genome. *Science, 226*, 1161–1165

98. Anderson, M.J., Lewis, E., Kidd, I.M., Hall, S.M. and Cohen, B.J., (1984). An outbreak of erythema infectiosum associated with human parvovirus infection. *J. Hyg. (Cambridge), 93*, 85–93

99. Reid, D.M., Reid, T.M.S., Brown, T., Rennie, J.A.N. and Eastmond, C.J. (1985). Human parvovirus-associated arthritis: a clinical and laboratory description. *Lancet, 1*, 422–425

100. Brown, T., Anand, A., Ritchie, L.D., Clewley, J.P. and Reid, T.M.S. (1984). Intrauterine parvovirus infection associated with hydrops fetalis. *Lancet,2*, 1033–1034

101. Anderson, M.J., Higgins, P.G., Davis, L.R., Williams, J.S., Jones, S.E., Kidd, I.M., Pattison, J.R. and Tyrrell, D.A.J. (1985). Experimental parvoviral infection in humans. *J. Infect. Dis., 152*, 257–265

102. Smith, C.A., Woolf, A.D. and Lenci, M. (1987). Parvoviruses: Infections and arthropathies. *Rheum. Dis. Clin. N. Am., 13*, 249–264

103. Clewley, J.P. (1985). Detection of human parvovirus using a molecularly cloned probe. *J. Med. Virol., 15*, 173–181

104. Luzzi, G.A., Kurtz, J.B. and Chapel, H. (1985). Human parvovirus arthropathy and rheumatoid factor. *Lancet, 1*, 1218

105. Lefrere, J.J., Meyer, O., Menkes, C.J., Beaulieu, M.M. and Courouce, A-M. (1985). Human parvovirus and rheumatoid arthritis. *Lancet, 1*, 982

106. Jones, V.E., Jacoby, R.K., Puttick, A.H. and Cohen, B.J. (1986). Rheumatoid arthritis; clinical onset, seropositivity and a possible cause. *Arthritis Rheum., 29*, 814–815

107. Duffy, J., Lidsky, M.D., Sharp, J.T., Davis, J.S., Person, D.A., Holliger, F.B. and Min, K.W. (1976). Polyarthritis, polyarteritis and hepatitis B. *Medicine (Baltimore), 55*, 19–37

108. Madhavan, T. and Cox, F. (1972). Anicteric hepatitis and polyathritis. *J. Am. Med. Assoc.* **220**, 1744–1745
109. Levo, Y., Gorevic, P. D., Kassab, H. J., Zucker-Franklin, D. and Franklin, E. C. (1977). Association between hepatitis B virus and essential mixed cryoglobulinaemia. *N. Engl. J. Med.*, **296**, 1501–1504
110. McCarty, D. J. and Ormiste, V. (1973). Arthritis and HB Ag-positive hepatitis. *Arch. Intern. Med.*, **132**, 264–268
111. Alpert, E., Isselbacher, K. J. and Schur, P. H. (1971). The pathogenesis of arthritis associated with viral hepatitis. *N. Engl. J. Med.*, **285**, 185–189
112. Koff, R. S. (1971). Immune-complex arthritis in viral hepatitis. *N. Engl. J. Med.*, **285**, 185–189
113. Dixon, F. J., Vasquez, J. J., Weigle, W. O. and Cochrane, C. G. (1958). Pathogenesis of serum sickness. *Arch. Pathol.*, **65**, 18
114. Orion, D. K., Crumpacker, C. S. and Gilliland, B. C. (1971). Arthritis of hepatitis associated with Australia antigen. *Ann. Intern. Med.*, **765**, 29–33
115. Wands, J. R., Mann, E., Alpert, E. and Isselbacher, K. J. (1975). The pathogenesis of arthritis associated with acute hepatitis B surface antigen-positive hepatitis. *J. Clin. Invest.*, **55**, 930–936
116. Rillet, M. (1850). Memoire sur une épidemie d'oreillons qui a regne a Geneve pendant les annees 1848 et 1849. *Gazette Médicale de Paris*, 22–25
117. ter Meulen, V. and Carter, M. J. (1982). Morbilliform persistent infections in animals and man. In Mahy, B. W. J., Minson, A. C. and Darby, G. K. (eds.) *Viral Persistence, 33rd Symposium Soc. Gen. Microbiol.* (Cambridge: Cambridge University Press)
118. Harvey, L. (1984). Viral aetiology of Paget's disease of bone: a review. *J. R. Soc. Med.*, **77**, 943–948
119. Maisondieu, P. (1924). Etude des manifestations articularies des orieillons. *Thèse pour le doctorat en médecine*, Paris, Jourve No. 519
120. Association for the Study of Infectious Diseases (1974). A retrospective survey of the complications of mumps. *J. R. Coll. Gen. Practit.*, **24**, 552–556
121. Gordan, S. C. and Lauter, C. B. (1984). Mumps arthritis: a review of the literature. *Rev. Infect. Dis.*, **6**, 338–343
122. Gold, H. E., Boxerbaum, B. and Leslie, H. J. Jr. (1968). Mumps arthritis. *Am. J. Dis. Child.*, **116**, 547–548
123. Gordan, S. C. and Lanter, C. B. (1982). Mumps arthritis: Unusual presentation as adult Still's disease. *Ann. Intern. Med.*, **97**, 45–47
124. Sigal, L. H., Steere, A. C. and Niederman, J. C. (1983). Symmetric polyarthritis associated with heterophile-negative infectious mononucleosis. *Arthritis Rheum.*, **26**, 553–556
125. Weiner, S. R. and Utsinger, P. D. (1988). Viral arthritis: a review with a description of 15 new cases. *Clin. Exp. Rheumatol.* (In press)
126. Ford, D. K., da Roza, D. M., Reid, G. D., Chantler, J. K. and Tingle, A. J. (1982). Synovial mononuclear cell responses to rubella antigen in rheumatoid arthritis and unexplained persistent knee arthritis. *J. Rheumatol.*, **9**, 420–423
127. Grahame, R., Armstrong, R., Simmons, N. A., Wilton, J. M. A., Dyson, M., Laurent, R., Mills, R. and Mims, C. A. (1983). Chronic arthritis associated with the presence of intrasynovial rubella virus. *Ann. Rheum. Dis.*, **42**, 2–13
128. Chantler, J. K., Tingle, A. J. and Petty, R. E. (1985). Persistent rubella virus

infection associated with chronic arthritis in children. *N. Engl. Med. J.*, **18**, 1117–1123

129. Simpson, R. W., McGinty, L., Simon, L., Smith, C. A., Godzeski, C. W. and Boyd, R. J. (1984). Association of parvoviruses with rheumatoid arthritis of humans. *Science*, **24**, 1425–1428

130. Alspaugh, M. A. and Tan, E. M. (1976). Serum antibody in rheumatoid arthritis reactive with a cell-associated antigen. *Arthritis Rheum.*, **19**, 711–719

131. Alspaugh, M. A., Jensen, F. C., Rabin, H. and Tan, E. M. (1978). Lymphocytes transformed by the Epstein–Barr virus. Induction of nuclear antigen reactive with antibody in rheumatoid arthritis. *J. Exp. Med.*, **147**, 1018–1027

132. Billings, P. B., Hoch, S. O., White, P. J., Carson, D. A. and Vaughan, J. H. (1983). Antibodies to Epstein–Barr virus nuclear antigen and to rheumatoid arthritis nuclear antigen identify the same polypeptide. *Proc. Natl. Acad. Sci.*, **80**, 7104–7108

133. Venables, P. J. W., Roffe, L. M., Erhardt, C. C. *et al.* (1981). Titres of antibodies of RANA in rheumatoid arthritis and normal sera. *Arthritis Rheum.*, **24**, 1459

134. Luka, J., Kreofsky, T., Pearson, G. R., Hennessy, K. and Keiff, E. (1984). Identification and characterisation of a cellular protein that cross-reacts with the Epstein–Barr virus nuclear antigen. *J. Virol.*, **52**, 833–838

135. Fox, R. I., Lotz, M., Rhodes, G. and Vaughan, J. H. (1985). Epstein–Barr virus in rheumatoid arthritis. *Clin. Rheum. Dis.*, **11**, 665–688

136. Depper, J. M., Bluestein, H. G. and Zvaigler, N. J. (1981). Impaired regulation of Epstein–Barr virus-induced lymphocyte proliferation in rheumatoid arthritis is due to a T cell defect. *J. Immunol.*, **127**, 1899–1902

137. Tosato, G., Steinberg, A. D. and Blaese, R. M. (1981). Defective EBV-specific suppressor T-cell function in rheumatoid arthritis. *N. Engl. J. Med.*, **305**, 1238–1243

138. Tosato, G., Steinberg, A. D., Yarchoan, R., Heilman, C. A., Pike, S. E., De Seau, V. and Blaese, R. M. (1984). Abnormally elevated frequency of Epstein–Barr virus-infected B cells in the blood of patients with rheumatoid arthritis. *J. Clin. Invest.*, **73**, 1789–1795

139. Stastny, P. (1978). Association of the B-cell alloantigen DRW4 with rheumatoid arthritis. *N. Engl. J. Med.*, **298**, 869–871

140. Panayi, G. S., Wooley, P. and Batchelor, J. R. (1978). Genetic basis of rheumatoid disease: HLA antigens, disease manifestations and toxic reactions to drugs. *Br. Med. J.*, **2**, 1326–1328

4

OPPORTUNISTIC ORGANISMS AND ARTHRITIS

P. W. THOMPSON

INTRODUCTION

In our world, micro-organisms are ubiquitous. The newborn are contaminated at birth and remain unknowing hosts to billions of microscopic parasites throughout life. Most are harmless commensals, some live in symbiosis, helping to digest food and furnishing vitamins, while others are pathogens causing disease.

Some pathogens are highly aggressive and are able to penetrate the defences of a normal healthy host (primary pathogens). Others are *opportunistic organisms* and only infect and cause disease if defence mechanisms have been broken.

Most of the time there is a balance between the pathogenic properties of the micro-organism and the defences of the host. Either is a potential aggressor against the other if the equilibrium is disturbed[1].

This chapter explores this balance of power.

ARTHRITIS AS A CAUSE OF OPPORTUNISTIC INFECTION

Chronic arthritis predisposes to infection. For example, there is no doubt that patients with rheumatoid arthritis[2] and systemic lupus erythematosus[3] (SLE) suffer more fatal infections than the normal population.

The predisposition is multifactorial. A combination of the disease process, its complications and treatment result in damage to superficial defences, and the humoral, phagocytic and cell-mediated immune mechanisms[4].

Any defect in the skin or mucous membrane will allow normal skin inhabitants to gain access to the body. Vasculitic ulcers, mouth ulcers in Behçet's disease or secondary to gold or D-penicillamine treatment, and pressure sores in the immobile arthritic patient are prone to superinfection with staphylococci and Gram-negative bacilli. There may be local abscess formation or septicaemia. The latter is a particular problem in hospitalized patients with indwelling catheters and intravenous lines.

Poorly perfused, damaged tissue offers an environment where opportunistic organisms can lodge and mutiply. The joint, damaged for whatever reason, is prone to chronic infection by micro-organisms which reach their target during transient bacteraemia (for example, following dental extraction).

Once past the superficial defences, pathogens encounter immunological mechanisms of protection, several of which may be defective because of the arthritic process or its treatment.

Although defects of humoral immunity are not characteristic of most inflammatory arthritic conditions[5], the rare complement deficiencies associated with lupus-like syndromes are associated with increased risk of infection. Patients receiving intensive immunosuppressive therapy may suffer immunoglobulin deficiency due to B-lymphocyte dysfunction, resulting in reduced bacterial opsonization and are prone to infections with encapsulated bacteria, such as pneumococci and *Haemophilus influenzae*.

Neutropenia occurs in Felty's syndrome and is a well-recognized side effect of second-line antirheumatoid drug therapy. There is an inverse relationship between the absolute peripheral neutrophil count and the risk of infection, so that, below $0.1 \times 10^{-9}/L$, almost all patients will acquire an infection[6]. Most infections occur in the lower respiratory tract, pharynx, perineum and urinary tract, and bacteraemia with no obvious portal of entry is common. Table 4.1 shows organisms which commonly cause infection in neutropenia[6].

Specific neutrophil disorders, such as Chediak–Higashi syndrome[7], are associated with an increased risk of infection. Similar, though less marked, defects in neutrophil function are well known in rheumatoid arthritis and SLE[5] and non-steroidal anti-inflammatory drugs have been shown to affect neutrophil chemotaxis[8], increasing the potential for opportunistic infection.

Defects in cell-mediated immunity are associated with increased risk of infection with tuberculosis, candida and herpes zoster. Such defects occur in rheumatoid arthritis and SLE[5].

Perhaps the chief culprits for the predisposition to infection are glucocorticoids, immunosuppressive drugs and total lymphoid irradiation. Table 4.2 lists some infections that occur in immuno-suppressed patients[9]. Infection is a particular risk when anti-proliferative drugs are given in combination with steroids[2].

It is surprising how infrequently infection results from the intra-articular injection of corticosteroids but the importance of such an event cannot be overemphasized. More common is the infection of an implanted prosthesis[10]. About a third of the latter infections occur via the blood following dental extractions or urinogenital instrumentation in the same way as chronic infections of damaged heart valves, and are caused by similar organisms, while two-thirds are introduced at the time of surgery. Table 4.3 shows a general view of the organisms commonly involved[10].

TABLE 4.1 Organisms commonly causing infection in neutropenia[6]

Gram-negative bacilli
Escherichia coli
Klebsiella
Pseudomonas aeruginosa
Serratia
Proteus
Enterobacter

Gram-positive bacilli
Staphylococcus aureus
Streptococcus pneumoniae
Group D streptococci

Fungi
Candida albicans
Aspergillus spp.

TABLE 4.2   Opportunistic organisms causing infection in immunosuppressive therapy[3]

Bacteria
Pyrogenic sepsis
Tuberculosis

Viruses
Herpes zoster
Varicella
Measles
Cytomegalovirus

Fungi
Candida
Coccidioidomycosis
Nocardia
Aspergillus
Cryptococcosis

Arthropodia
Scabies

TABLE 4.3   Organisms causing infection in prosthetic joints[10]

Staphylococci
Epidermis
Aureus

Streptococci
Pyogenes (group A)
Agalactiae (Group B)
Faecalis (enterococcus)

Gram-negative bacilli

Anaerobes

OPPORTUNISTIC ORGANISMS AS A CAUSE OF CHRONIC ARTHRITIS

It may be interesting to look at things from the other direction and consider how those organisms which are frequently associated with opportunistic infection may produce arthritis in normal individuals.

The causative associations between micro-organisms and arthritis may be considered as occurring in four ways[11] (Table 4.4).

Infective arthritis[2]

Septic arthritis may arise spontaneously or may supervene in rheumatoid arthritis, mechanically damaged joints (including neuropathic joints), in debilitating disease, and following immunosuppressive therapy.

Tuberculous arthritis is of increasing importance in immigrant populations in the UK. It frequently arises in an otherwise fit individual and may occur several years after arrival in this country. It may affect any joint.

Bone and joint infection with histoplasmosis is very rare in the UK but an important cause of infection in the Americas. Arthralgia may accompany the rash of erythema nodosum or multiforme which sometimes occurs in association with pulmonary histoplasmosis in a similar way to pulmonary tuberculosis.

Occasionally a polyarthritis is associated with overwhelming systemic infection with toxoplasma, cytomegalovirus, herpes zoster or listeria.

Rarely, a prosthetic joint will become chronically infected following haematogenous spread from a primary infection with fungi, such as candida, nocardia or aspergillus.

Infection with pneumocystis or herpes simplex is not usually associated with arthritis.

TABLE 4.4 Possible causal relationship between infective organisms and arthritis[11]

Class	Agent known	Viable organism in joint	Non-viable organism in joint	Arthritic syndrome
I	+	+	+	Infective
II	+	−	+	Post-infective
III	+	−	−	Reactive
IV	−	−	−	Inflammatory

Post-infective arthritis

Although, strictly speaking, not opportunistic pathogens, the meningococci and gonococci are capable of producing an arthritis during the recovery phase of systemic infection. In the majority of these cases, the synovial fluid is sterile but bacterial antigen–antibody immune complexes can be found in the synovium associated with chronic inflammatory cells and the arthritis is likely to be the result of an Arthus reaction[12].

Reactive arthritis

The Group A β-haemolytic streptococcus commonly produces upper respiratory tract infections which are complicated by rheumatic fever in a few cases. It may be thought of as an opportunistic organism, producing articular disease in susceptible hosts. The cause of the arthritis is uncertain but anti-connective tissue antibodies have been detected and it may be an example of a cross-reactive antibody phenomenon[13].

Several other examples of reactive arthritis are known to the rheumatologist although the same clinical picture can be produced by several different organisms. The gut-associated and sexually-acquired reactive arthritides are examples and have been linked with infections with salmonella, shigella, yersinia and campylobacter in the former, and chlamydia and ureaplasma in the latter[14].

Inflammatory arthritis

What of the chronic inflammatory arthritides where evidence for an association with an infective organism has not been forthcoming? Diphtheroids[15], mycoplasma[16], viruses[17],[18] and many other organisms have been put forward as causative organisms in rheumatoid arthritis, and klebsiella, among several gut opportunists, as the cause of ankylosing spondylitis. To date, there is no convincing evidence that an individual organism is implicated. It may be that the host is genetically susceptible to the production of arthritis following infection with a variety of micro-organisms. If this is the case, then chronic arthritis would be the result of, as well as a cause of, infection with opportunistic organisms!

REFERENCES

1. Frobisher, M., Hinsdill, R. D., Crabtree, K. T. and Goodheart, C. R. (1974). *Fundamentals of Microbiology*, 9th Edn., pp. 332–333. (Philadelphia: WB Saunders)
2. Scott, D. L. and Symmons, D. P. M. (1986). The mortality of rheumatoid arthritis. In *Reports on Rheumatic Diseases* (*Series 2*) (London: Arthritis and Rheumatism Council)
3. Helve, T. (1985). Prevalence and mortality rates of systemic lupus erythematosus and cause of death in SLE patients in Finland. *Scand. J. Rheumatol.*, **14**, 43–46
4. Dale, D. C. (1980). Infections in the compromised host. In Isselbacher, K. J, Adams, R. D., Braunwald, E., Petersdorf, R. G. and Wilson, J. D. (eds.) *Harrison's Principles of Internal Medicine*, 9th Edn., pp. 552–556. (New York: McGraw-Hill)
5. Lockshin, M. D. (1976). Immunological status of patients with rheumatic disease. In Dumonde, D. C. (ed.) *Infection and Immunology in the Rheumatic Diseases*, pp. 541–547. (Oxford: Blackwell)
6. Ronald, A. R. and Riben, P. D. (1981). Infections in the immunocompromised host. *Med. Int.*, **2**, 39–43
7. Wintrobe, M. M. (1974). *Clinical Haematology*, 7th Edn. (Philadelphia: Lea and Febiger)
8. Abramson, S., Edelson, H., Kaplan, H., Ludewig, R. and Weissmann, G. (1984). Inhibition of neutrophil activation by non-steroidal anti-inflammatory drugs. *Am. J. Med.*, **77** (4B), 3–6
9. Currey, H. L. F. (1983). Drugs affecting the immune response. In Holborow, E. J. and Reeves, W. G. (eds.) *Immunology in Medicine*, 2nd Edn., pp. 1589–611. (London, New York: Academic Press)
10. Brause, B. D. (1986). Infection associated with prosthetic joints. *Clin. Rheum. Dis.*, **12**, 523–536
11. Dumonde, D. C. (ed.) (1976). *Infection and Immunology in the Rheumatic Diseases*, p. 96. (Oxford: Blackwell)
12. Greenwood, B. M. and Whittle, H. C. (1976). The pathogenesis of meningococcal arthritis. In Dumonde, D. C. (ed.) *Infection and Immunology in the Rheumatic Diseases*, pp. 119–132. (Oxford: Blackwell)
13. Zabriskie, J. B. (1976). Rheumatic fever: a streptococcal induced auto-immune disease? In Dumonde, D. C. (ed.) *Infection and Immunology in the Rheumatic Diseases*, pp. 97–111. (Oxford: Blackwell)
14. Ford, D. K. (1986). Reactive arthritis: a viewpoint rather than a review. *Clin. Rheum. Dis.*, **12**, 389–401
15. Duthie, J. J. R., Stewart, S. M. and McBride, W. H. (1976). Do diptheroids cause rheumatoid arthritis? In Dumonde, D. C. (ed.) *Infection and Immunology in the Rheumatic Diseases*, pp. 171–175. (Oxford: Blackwell)

16. Taylor-Robinson, D. and Taylor, G. (1976). Do mycoplasmas cause rheumatic disease? In Dumonde, D. C. (ed.) *Infection and Immunology in Rheumatic Diseases*, pp. 177–186. (Oxford: Blackwell)
17. Mamion, B. P. (1976). A microbiologist's view of investigative rheumatology. In Dumonde, D. C. (ed.) *Infection and Immunology in the Rheumatic Diseases*, pp. 245–258. (Oxford: Blackwell)
18. White, D. G.. Woolf, A. D., Mortimer, P. P., Cohen, B. J., Blake, D. R. and Bacon, P. A. (1985). Human parvovirus arthropathy. *Lancet*, **1**, 419–421

5
ARTHRITIS IN LEPROSY AND SCHISTOSOMIASIS

S. L. ATKIN

INTRODUCTION

Leprosy and schistosomiasis are chronic infectious diseases which have afflicted mankind since the days of antiquity and indeed both are referred to in the Quran. They are a major cause of disability and, despite advances in chemotherapy, there is evidence to show that far from being historic diseases on the decline, in fact, their prevalence is increasing. Apart from the morbidity and mortality of the diseases, they impose a major economic burden on developing countries in terms of lost manpower, treatment and rehabilitation, further stretching the overextended health services.

One need look no further than the socioeconomic impact of arthritis in patients in developed countries to see the effect of arthritis superimposed upon the backcloth of the manifestations of leprosy and schistosomiasis.

SCHISTOSOMIASIS AND ARTHRITIS

Schistosomiasis (bilharziasis) is a group of diseases mainly affecting the genitourinary and gastrointestinal systems. It is caused by a trematode of the genus *Schistosoma*, of which the three most common species to affect man are *S. mansoni*, *S. haematobium* and *S. japonicum*. Each tends to afflict a different geographical and ethnic group. Even within one country, different forms are prevalent in different regions[1].

The life cycles of the three species are similar. Arthritis has only been described in schistosomiasis in Egypt to date and therefore the discussion will be restricted to *S. mansoni* and *S. haematobium*, which are both endemic to that country[1]. Man is the definitive host and is infected by contact with fresh slow-running water containing schistosome cercariae. The cercariae penetrate the skin, develop into tailless schistosomules and actively migrate throughout the body to localize selectively in small terminal blood vessels. Most adult *S. haematobium* live in the prostatic, bladder and uterine venous plexuses, whereas *S. mansoni* inhabit the venules of the inferior mesenteric plexus of the portal tract. They lie in intimate contact as paired adults. Following fertilization, the ova are released from the bladder (*S. haematobium*) and the intestine (*S. mansoni*) and hatch immediately in fresh water to free-swimming miricidiae. The miricidiae infect a specific snail secondary host in which, following two sporocyst generations, they develop into cercariae to repeat the cycle of infection. The prevalence of schistosomiasis in Egypt has increased dramatically since the construction of the Aswan Dam, to become epidemic throughout lower Egypt[2].

An arthritis associated with *S. mansoni* infection was first documented in 1966[3]. Patients with active schistosomiasis infection presenting with conspicuous back, knee and ankle pain was described. Bassiouni and Kamel[4] noted a similar distribution of arthritis in patients with active schistosomiasis infection affecting the heels (41%), sacroiliac joints (41%), cervical spine (30%), knees (27%), dorsal spine (21%) and tarsal joints (4%). X-ray appearances of the cervicodorsal spine, knees, hands and feet were all within normal limits. However, the sacroiliac and heel X-rays showed pathological changes of 'an inflammatory character.' The heels showed plantar fasciitis and an Achilles tendonitis, calcaneal spurs and periosteal reactions were seen. The sacroiliac joints showed loss of articular margins, erosions and widening. Synovial biopsy revealed ova in the synovium in three patients with a surrounding reactive synovitis. Knee arthroscopy and open surgery in others with arthritis showed reactive changes within the synovium devoid of ova. Rheumatoid factor was positive in 3% of patients and it was concluded that X-ray changes of the heels and sacroiliac joints were of diagnostic value. In both studies[3,4], there was

94

neither morning stiffness nor inactivity stiffness. Articular swelling and synovial effusion were not described.

In a study of 96 patients with active *S. mansoni* infection only, 72 patients with prominent musculoskeletal complaints were described. Nine patients presented with a peripheral polyarthritis alone, 16 patients had an enthesitis alone and 47 were suffering from a combination of both an arthritis and an enthesitis. The patients with musculoskeletal disease were significantly older and the length of exposure to recurrent infections with schistosomiasis was greater than in those patients with schistosomiasis alone. The arthritis was peripheral and symmetrical in distribution in 42 patients, affecting the proximal interphalangeal and metacarpophalangeal joints, wrists, knees and ankles. In 21 patients, the arthritis was pauciarticular (less than four joints affected) in distribution with a similar joint predilection in a variable combination. All of the patients with a pauciarticular arthritis had a concomitant enthesitis. The enthesitis affected those sites of insertion into the nuchal crest, the shoulder, the medial and lateral epicondyles of the elbow, the iliac crests and pubic symphysis, the femoral tubercles, sites of insertion into and out of the patella and into the tibial tubercle, sites of insertion of the medial and lateral collateral ligaments of the knee, site of insertion of the Achilles tendon and of the plantar aponeurosis. The enthesitis was not localized to any particular site or distribution.

The musculoskeletal symptoms presented three days to two weeks after the first symptoms of schistosomiasis infection, with joint pain alone or in combination with pain at the site of the enthesis. Prominent morning stiffness, lasting 30 minutes to 2 hours, and marked inactivity stiffness, lasting up to 30 minutes, was described. The joints were tender and warm, but not red, with soft-tissue swelling due to synovial effusions. There was related muscle atrophy.

Synovial fluid taken from 4 patients revealed an inflammatory picture and bacterial culture was negative. Unfortunately, no synovial biopsies were taken. Radiology of the affected joints was unremarkable, with no evidence of an underlying erosive process. The acute phase reactant α-1-acid glycoprotein was found to 'mark' those patients with arthritis, being lowered significantly.

IgM rheumatoid factor was noted in 5 patients with schistosomiasis with arthritis but also in 4 patients without schistosomiasis without

95

arthritis[5]. Seropositivity for IgM rheumatoid factor has been previously documented in schistosomiasis[6,7], restricting the value of this investigation in establishing or excluding rheumatoid arthritis. In two studies[3,5], the musculoskeletal symptoms resolved on specific anti-schistosomiasis medication, with little response to corticosteroids or to non-steroidal anti-inflammatory drugs. Eight patients are described[5] where musculoskeletal symptoms completely resolved within one month of instituting medication with a further 2 suffering continuing symptoms after this period. Males and females appear to be affected equally.

It would be unusual for the two types of arthritis described in patients with schistosomiasis, affecting the back and large joints of the lower limbs[3,4] and in a peripheral distal distribution[5] with an enthesitis, to remain clinically distinct entities. Further research will probably find that there is a range of musculoskeletal presentations in these patients.

LEPROSY AND ARTHRITIS

Leprosy is a disease caused by the obligate intracellular parasite, *Mycobacterium leprae*[8]. WHO estimate that there are 10.8 million cases and, of these, about 18% are under treatment[9]. Depending upon the strength of the cellular immune response against *M. leprae*, a spectrum of clinical presentations may result[10]. Patients may be classified according to Ridley and Jopling[8] by a combination of clinical and histopathological features into determinate and indeterminate forms. The determinate patients may be divided into tuberculoid leprosy (TT), borderline tuberculoid (BT), borderline (BB), borderline lepromatous (BL) and lepromatous leprosy (LL). Borderline patients (BT–BL) change their classification, while patients with polar disease tend not to shift. Those patients with high resistance, i.e. well-developed cell-mediated immunity to *M. leprae*, develop tuberculoid leprosy in which the disease is localized to the skin and peripheral nerves, whereas those with low resistance develop lepromatous leprosy, in which generalized infection develops.

Bacilli are shed in the order of 10^7 to 10^8 per day from the nasal mucosa of LL patients and inhalation is the most probable method of infection[11].

The incubation period is measured in years and may become manifest decades after leaving an infected area.

Neuropathic or Charcot's joints are mentioned in all descriptions in the major textbooks of leprosy and rheumatology. Lepra Type II or erythema nodosum leprosum (ENL) reactions are likewise found in all major texts[12,13]. ENL reactions occur predominantly in LL and, to a lesser extent, BL. They may occur spontaneously or may be provoked by intercurrent infection, stress, injury or surgery, immunization, pregnancy or parturition. Systemic disturbance may be marked with red painful skin nodules, superficial or deep to the dermis, nerve pain, bone pain, rhinitis, epistaxis, acute iridiocyclitis, swollen and tender lymphadenopathy, acute epididymal orchitis, proteinuria and arthritis. The arthritis, with or without joint swelling, occurs following the onset of the constitutional symptoms and signs of ENL with day-to-day variation in severity[14]. The joints affected are those of the shoulders, elbows, knees, ankles and small joints of the hands and feet. Several joints may be affected together from the onset, or joints may be sequentially involved. Joint swelling is due to synovial effusions, aspiration of which shows an inflammatory reaction but bacterial culture is negative. The acute joint changes resolve leaving no residual disability. ENL reactions are thought to be due to an 'Arthus' reaction where there is a reactive arthropathy to precipitating immune complexes in the tissues[15]. Thalidomide, 100–400 mg per day, is the drug of choice except in premenopausal women. Alternatively, reducing doses of prednisolone, commencing at 30 mg per day, or clofazimine, initially 300 mg per day, may be used. Clofazimine may be used to wean patients off steroids who are troubled with continuous ENL and where thalidomide cannot be used. Clofazimine may temporarily aggravate reactions and therefore should be given under steroid cover.

It has been suggested that leprosy is a disease which is analogous in many ways to rheumatoid arthritis[16]. Albert, Weisman and Kaplan[17] examined 21 patients and documented erythema nodosum with and without arthritis in 5 and 9 patients respectively, 'swollen hand syndrome' in 3 patients and single patients with 'dermatomyositis-like' disease and vasculitis. In a clinical abstract[18], 18 unselected leprosy patients were examined, 14 of whom were without ENL reactions, had chronic episodic pain, swelling and impairment of function affecting several large joints (wrists, elbows and knees), and small joints (hands), but there is little detailed description of the affected joint distribution. Radiological erosions were noted but there is no indication of their site. Synovial biopsies in 4 patients showed oedema and lymphocytic infiltration but no acid-fast bacilli were demonstrated. Similarly, in two large-scale studies from India[19,20], it is reported that musculo-skeletal manifestations were encountered in a proportion of patients but few details were given.

More recently, a clinical and radiological study of 66 leprosy patients[14] documented a peripheral symmetrical polyarthritis in 20 patients and arthritis in 12 patients with ENL reactions together with one patient with lucio phenomenon–necrotizing ENL[21].

The symmetrical peripheral polyarthritis affected the wrists, meta-carpal and proximal interphalangeal joints of the hands, the knees and metatarsophalangeal joints of the feet. The arthritis evolved months or years after the onset of the first symptoms of leprosy and appeared independently of ENL or lepra Type I reactions. The onset was insidious with a pattern of exacerbations and remissions. Morning stiffness and inactivity stiffness were conspicuous. All of the patients suffered from joint swelling due to synovial effusion and swelling, tenderness over the joint margin and pain in both active and passive movements of the joints. The arthritis responded poorly to non-steroidal anti-inflammatory agents but appeared to respond to anti-leprosy medication. The authors were unable to say whether this was due to the natural history of the arthritis or the influence of medication. In some, permanent structural deformities, such as swan neck, bou-tonniere and trigger finger deformity were noted. The arthritis was erosive in 11 patients, affecting the carpal bones, metacarpophalangeal and proximal interphalangeal joints of the hands and the meta-tarsophalangeal joints of the feet. The destructive arthritis did not differ in clinical presentation or evolution within any leprosy subgroup. However, the study was unable to determine whether those patients with arthritis without erosions would have progressed to a destructive stage.

IgM rheumatoid factor[14] was found more commonly in those patients without arthritis than those with arthritis. IgM rheumatoid

98

factor is commonly found in leprosy[7,22] restricting the value of the investigation and confirming or excluding rheumatoid arthritis, an observation similar to that of the arthritis in schistosomiasis.

PUTATIVE MECHANISMS

The aetiology of the arthritis found in both schistosomiasis and leprosy is unclear. Ova have been documented in the synovium in schistosomiasis[4], and 'lepra' cells (macrophages filled with replicating *M. leprae* bacilli) have been found in the synovial fluid of a leprosy patient[17]. It is possible that the arthritis associated with both leprosy and schistosomiasis is being initiated by, and is perpetuated by, the respective organisms. In the event of this explanation being correct, then the questions will arise: is the synovitis produced directly by the presence of replicating organisms in the synovium? is the synovitis the result of the presence of microbial antigen in synovium? or is the synovitis the result locally of the presence elsewhere in the body of the microbial antigen? The identification of the underlying mechanisms responsible for the joint inflammation in these diseases may offer enhanced insight into diseases of unknown aetiology, such as rheumatoid arthritis.

In both leprosy and schistosomiasis, arthritis may be the presenting complaint of the diseases[5,14]. Although the general practitioner or rheumatologist in the developed country is unlikely to meet either disease, in a world of rapid air travel and an immigrant population there must be an awareness of leprosy and schistosomiasis, albeit low in a differential diagnosis of patients presenting with arthritis.

REFERENCES

1. Khalil, H. M. (1978). Schistosomiasis in Egypt. *J. Egypt. Public Health Assoc.*, **53**, 67–86
2. Abdel-Wahab, M. F., El Sahly, A., Zakaria, S., Strickland, G. T., El-Kady, N. and Ahmed, L. (1979). Changing patterns of schistosomiasis in Egypt 1935–79. *Lancet*, **1**, 242–244
3. Girges, M. R. (1966). Schistosomal arthritis. *Rheumatism*, **22** (4), 108

4. Bassiouni, M. and Kamel, M. (1984) Bilharzial arthropathy. *Ann. Rheum. Dis.*, **43**, 806–809
5. Atkin, S. L., Kamel, M., El-Hady, A. M. A., El-Badawy, S. A., El-Ghobary, A. and Dick, W. C. (1986). Schistosomiasis and inflammatory polyarthritis: A clinical, radiological and laboratory study of 96 patients infected by *S.mansoni* with particular reference to the diarthrodial joint. *Q. J. Med.*, **59**, 479–487
6. Carvahlo, E. M., Andrews, B. S., Martinelli, R., Dutra, M. and Rocha, H. (1983). Circulating immune complexes and rheumatoid factor in schistosomiasis and visceral leishmaniasis. *Am. J. Trop. Med. Hyg.*, **32** (1), 61–68
7. Gonzales-Pares, E. N., Franco, A. E., De La Cruz, S., Molares, F. R., Gonzales-Alcover, R. and Bryan, R. M. (1973). False positive latex in a tropical area. *J. Chron. Dis.*, **26**, 31–38
8. Ridley, D. S. and Jopling, W. H. (1966). Classification of leprosy according to immunity: A five group system. *Int. J. Lep.*, **34**, 255–273
9. World Health Organisation (1977). *Fifth Report of the WHO Expert Committee on Leprosy*. Section 1:1 Tech. Rep. Ser. No. 607, Geneva
10. Myrvang, B., Godal, T., Ridley, ⟨D. S., Froland, S. S. and Song, Y. K. (1973). Immune responsiveness to *Mycobacterium leprae* and other mycobacterial antigens throughout the clinical and histological spectrum of leprosy. *Clin. Exp. Immunol.*, **14**, 541–543
11. Bryceson, A. and Pfaltzgraff, R. E. (1979). Epidemilogy. In *Leprosy*, 2nd Edn., Chapt. 14, pp. 126–135. (Edinburgh, London and New York: Churchill Livingstone)
12. Jopling, W. M. (1971). *Handbook of Leprosy*, pp. 44–62. (London: William Heinneman Medical Books Ltd)
13. Karat, A. B. A., Karat, S. and Job, C. K. (1966). Acute exudative arthritis in leprosy: rheumatoid-arthritis like syndrome in association with erythema nodosum leprosum. *Br. Med. J.*, **3**, 770–773
14. Atkin (submitted for publication)
15. Sharma, V. K., Saha, K. and Sehgal, V. N. (1982). Serum immunglobulins and autoantibodies during and after erythema nodosum leprosum (ENL). *Int. J. Lep.*, **50** (2), 159–163
16. Panayi, G. S. (1982). Viewpoint: does rheumatoid arthritis have a clinicopathological similarity to leprosy? *Ann. Rheum. Dis.*, **41**, 102–103
17. Albert, D. A., Weissman, M. H. and Kaplan, R. (1980). The rheumatic manifestations of leprosy (Hansen's disease). *Medicine*, **59**, 442–448
18. Alcocer, J. V., Herrera, C. L., Gudino, J. and Fraga, A. (1979). Inflammatory arthropathy in leprosy. *Arthritis Rheum.*, **22**, , 597 (abstract)
19. Lele, R. C., Sainani, G. S. and Sharma, K. D. (1965). Leprosy presenting as rheumatoid arthritis. *J. Assoc. Phys. India*, **13**, 275
20. Medi, T. H. and Lele, R. C. (1969). Acute joint manifestations in leprosy. *J. Assoc. Phys. India*, **17**, 247
21. Frenken, J. H. (1963). *Diffuse Leprosy of Lucio and Latapi*. (Detroit: Blaine Ethridge)
22. Cathcart, E. S., Williams, R. C., Ross, S. H. *et al.* (1962). The relationship of the latex fixation test to the clinical and serological manifestations of leprosy. *Am. J. Med.*, **56**, 545–552
23. Louie, J. S., Koransky, J. R. and Cohen, A. H. (1973). Lepra cells in synovial fluid of a patient with erythema nodosum leprosum. *N. Engl. J. Med.*, **289**, 1410

6
ARBOVIRUS ARTHRITIS

D. WALKER

INTRODUCTION

Many virus infections are associated with the development of an arthritis. In Britain and the USA, common associations are with hepatitis B, mumps and rubella, whilst, in other parts of the world, arboviruses are implicated in the pathogenesis of joint disease.

The term arbovirus is a contraction of the phrase arthropod-borne virus. Arboviruses are defined by the WHO as 'viruses which are maintained in nature principally, or to an important extent, through biological transmission between susceptible vertebrate hosts by haematophagous arthropods; they multiply and produce viraemia in vertebrates, multiply in the tissues of arthropods and are passed on to new vertebrates by the bite of an arthropod after a period of extrinsic incubation'. This definition excludes viruses which are merely transferred mechanically between vertebrates by insects. The arboviruses are remarkable for their ability to reproduce in both arthropod and mammalian cells.

The classification of a virus as an arbovirus is based on its mode of transmission and is unrelated to the morphological or functional characteristics of the virus, or to the clinical syndrome with which it is associated. Arboviruses are drawn from several families, notably Togaviridae, Arenaviridae, Bunyaviridae, Reoviridae and Rhabdoviridae, and from many genera which are determined serologically[1].

The concept of viruses as the causative agents of disease was developed from the observations of Ivanowsky, who showed in 1892 that tobacco mosaic disease was caused by material which could be passed through a fine-pore filter. The phenomenon of disease transmission by true arthropod vectors was first demonstrated by Manson in 1878, who described transmission of the filiarial worm, *Wuchereria bancrofti*, by mosquito vector. This was followed by the demonstration by Ross of transmission of the malarial parasite by mosquitos.

The first arbovirus to be described was yellow fever virus. This disease was shown to be transmissable by mosquito vector by Walter Reed in 1901 after extensive studies of the condition amongst American servicemen in Cuba. It was confirmed to be a filterable virus by Stokes *et al.* in 1927. In the sixty years since then, over 400 arboviruses have been described of which more than 100 are associated with disease in man.

The arboviruses constitute a vast heterogeneous group of organisms. It is not surprising that arbovirus infections are associated with a broad spectrum of clinical syndromes. Encephalitic and haemorrhagic syndromes are described following infection with specific groups of arboviruses. Many arbovirus infections are associated with non-specific symptoms, or diagnosed only after investigation for pyrexia of unknown origin. A small group of arboviruses produce a clinical syndrome of which joint symptoms are the major complaint. This group is the subject of this chapter.

The principal members of this group are Ross river, Chikungunya, Sindbis and O'nyong nyong. These viruses share a common basic structure. They are single-stranded RNA viruses of icosahedral shape enclosed in a lipid envelope. They are all classified in the family Togaviridae and the genus *Alphavirus*, although arthritis associated with viruses classified in other genera is now being recognized. The clinical syndromes associated with infection by these viruses are very similar but the epidemiology and ecology of the viruses are quite diffferent.

All of these viruses are transmitted by mosquito vectors. The virus is present in the saliva of the mosquito and is introduced into the host by the bite of the mosquito. If the virus is able to multiply, a viraemia occurs several days later which coincides with the onset of symptoms. Antibodies to the virus appear in the blood 2–4 days after the onset of symptoms. High titres of these antibodies may persist for many years[2]. The patient retains lifelong immunity to that particular virus type. This immunity may not protect the individual from different serotypes of that virus. In the pathogenesis of Dengue fever, a group B arbovirus, it has been suggested that second infection by a different serotype may result in the much more severe haemorrhagic form of the disease. This may be due to antibody to the first type combining with the second virus without neutralizing it. Virus entry to host cells might then be facilitated by interaction between antibody and host cell Fc receptors[3].

ACUTE ARTHRITIS ASSOCIATED WITH ARBOVIRUS INFECTION

Chikungunya

The name Chikungunya is derived from the Swahili words meaning 'that which bends joints up'. Chikungunya infection occurs in epidemics with sporadic cases occurring between epidemics. The mechanism of virus survival between epidemics is unclear. The virus was first isolated[4] after an epidemic in Tanzania in 1952–3. Epidemics have since been described in South Africa, Nigeria, India, Cambodia, Thailand and Zimbabwe. Historical evidence suggests that many epidemics described prior to 1953, previously ascribed to Dengue virus, were in fact Chikungunya[5].

African studies implicate wild primates, including vervet monkeys and baboons, as the principal hosts other than man[6]. Transmission studies have shown that the virus can be transmitted readily by several mosquitos of the genera *Aedes* and *Mansonia*[7,8]. The principal African vector is *Aedes furcifer-taylori* although *Aedes aegypti* has been implicated in urban epidemics.

After infection with Chikungunya, there is an incubation period of 2–19 days. This is followed by an acute onset of fever, headache, rigors, arthralgia, myalgia, nausea, vomiting and diarrhoea. A skin rash develops on the trunk, limbs, palms and soles of the feet which is of maculopapular or morbilliform appearance. The skin rash may fade and reappear several times during the acute phase of the disease. Photophobia and lymphadenopathy may be present. The fever, headache, rash and gastrointestinal symptoms resolve spontaneously over 2–7 days[9,10].

The most striking feature of Chikungunya infection is severe joint pain. The articular manifestations typically appear 3–5 days after onset of the first symptoms. The most commonly affected joints are the MCP joints, wrists, elbows, shoulders, knees, ankles and MTP joints. Joint involvement is symmetrical. Any synovial joint may be involved, particularly previously injured joints. The hip is not commonly affected. The affected joints are swollen, stiff and painful even at rest. Pain is exacerbated by overexertion of the joint[11]. Symptoms are less severe in children and resolve more quickly.

In most cases, the articular symptoms regress and disappear over a period of 1–12 months. Occasionally, the joint symptoms do not resolve and the condition becomes chronic.

Sindbis

Sindbis virus was first isolated in the Sindbis region of the Nile delta in Egypt[12]. The virus has since been isolated in Africa, Southern Asia, Czechoslovakia, USSR and Australia. The principal hosts other than man are wild birds[13]. Sindbis virus has been isolated from many species of mosquito, particularly of the genus *Culex*. Human infection tends to occur sporadically despite a high prevalence of the virus in other hosts in some areas. This may be due to a high incidence of subclinical infection, or to a low biting rate on man of the vector species.

Infection with Sindbis presents after an incubation period of 2–5 days with a prodrome of mild fever, malaise, headache and generalized joint and muscle pains. A rash then develops on the trunk and limbs. The rash is usually maculopapular and pruritic. Vesicles may develop on hands and feet. The rash tends to disappear from limbs and trunk in the order in which it appeared[14]. Joint pain and swelling are common and may be severe. Stiffness may also be present. The joints most commonly affected are the small joints of hands and feet[15]. The symptoms usually disappear in 10–14 days but residual joint pain may occur.

O'nyong nyong

O'nyong nyong virus was first described during an epidemic of a dengue-like illness which began in Uganda in 1959[1]. O'nyong nyong in the local dialect means 'joint-breaker'. The epidemic spread throughout Kenya, Malawi and Tanzania[1].

The principal vertebrate hosts other than man have yet to be described. Arboviruses are mainly transmitted by culicine mosquitos, particularly of the genera *Culex* and *Aedes*. In the East African epidemic, the insect vectors were anophelines, principally *Anopheles funestus* and *Anopheles gambiae*[1].

The documented clinical descriptions of O'nyong nyong fever were all produced by the East African Virus Research Institute during the 1959 epidemic. The onset of O'nyong nyong fever was typically sudden. The incubation period was probably greater than eight days. The principal symptom was joint pain. The joints most commonly affected were wrists, elbows, knees, ankles and the small joints of the hands. A morbilliform rash appeared after three to four days. Lymphadenopathy was present and usually a prominent feature of the illness. Headache and low-grade fever were almost universally present[16,17].

O'nyong nyong is very similar to Chikungunya, both antigenically, in that antibodies to the virus raised in humans will cross-react with Chikungunya virus, and in the clinical syndrome with which it is associated. Certainly these viruses may be distinguished serologically but the degree of antigenic overlap suggests that O'nyong nyong may be an antigenic variant of Chikungunya[18].

Ross river

A syndrome of polyarthralgia and rash occurring in epidemics was first described in Australia by Nimmo in 1928[19]. The syndrome became known as 'epidemic polyarthritis'. Patients with the syndrome were shown to have high antibody titres to Ross river virus[20]. The virus was finally isolated from patients with the syndrome in 1971[21]. The condition is endemic in Australia and several hundred cases are diagnosed every year in Australia. The condition has also been reported

105

in New Guinea and the Solomon Islands. Recent epidemics of many thousands of cases have been reported in Fiji and American Samoa.

In the pacific island epidemics, the high incidence of antibodies to the virus in humans compared with other vertebrates suggested that the virus was maintained in a mosquito–man–mosquito cycle. In Australia, the disease is endemic and wild vertebrates are important hosts other than man. The principal vectors in Australia are thought to be *Culex annulirostris* and *Aedes vigilax*. Ross river virus has been shown to cross the placenta in humans[22].

The incubation period is 7–9 days[23]. The low clinical infection rate may be due to clearance or inactivation of the virus during this period by non-specific immunological mechanisms in non-susceptible individuals[24]. The principal clinical features are fever, sore throat, maculopapular or vesicular rash and polyarthralgia. The joints most commonly involved are the small joints of hands and feet. Effusions and joint swelling may occur. The symptoms usually subside in days or weeks but joint pain persist for years[25].

Other arboviruses

Many other arboviruses are associated with arthritis. Mayaro is a group A arbovirus which is found on the American continent[26]. Infection may result in fever and joint pain with or without swelling. Mayaro tends to occur during yellow fever epidemics. This is probably due to both viruses being transmitted by the same mosquito vectors of the genus *Haemogogus*. The principal hosts other than man are thought to be wild primates[27].

West Nile, Dengue and Igbo-Ora viruses are all reported to cause arthritis in some cases. Early reports have to led to some confusion between these viruses and Chikungunya or Sindbis due to similarities in epidemiology or clinical features[15,18], or inadequate diagnostic techniques.

CHRONIC ARTHRITIS ASSOCIATED WITH ARBOVIRUS INFECTION

It has been noted by many authors that the arthritis associated with arboviruses does not always resolve with the disappearance of the other symptoms of acute infection. Joint pain, swelling and stiffness may persist for months or years.

There are sporadic reports of subacute or chronic arthritis following infection with Sindbis, Ross river and West Nile viruses.

In a retrospective study of 117 patients presenting with epidemic polyarthritis in Queensland, Australia, 20 replies were received to a questionnaire concerning persistence of joint pains. Of these, 6 reported persistence of joint symptoms, particularly of the feet and ankles[28].

Chronic arthritis following Chikungunya infection is documented more comprehensively. A study of 20 patients in the acute phase of Chikungunya infection and four months after the acute phase, was conducted in 1980[29]. At four months, 15% were suffering severe pain, 45% were still symptomatic and 40% were suffering little or no pain. A mean duration of morning stiffness of 62.5 minutes was recorded with only 2 patients free of this symptom. Grip strength was below normal in 90% of patients. Radiographs showed some soft tissue swelling in 40% and revealed 2 small erosions in the MCP joints of 1 patient. No control radiographs were available and so the abnormal features cannot be assumed to be a result of Chikungunya infection. Three patients had raised serum acute-phase protein levels and 2 developed positive rheumatoid factor titres.

In a study of 28 patients with Chikungunya infection, 5 patients had persistent symptoms 20 months after onset of symptoms[9]. No radiological abnormalities were present 1 year after onset of symptoms.

In a retrospective study of 107 patients, all of whom had contracted acute Chikungunya infection 40–60 months previously, 88% recovered completely after a variable period of up to 3 years. A further 6% had occasional or persistent joint symptoms. The principal symptoms were morning stiffness, gelling after rest and mild pain. The remaining 6% had persistent severe pain and stiffness. Some had joint swelling. Effusions were common. The most commonly affected joints were the wrists, ankles, knees, MCP and MTP joints. Radiographs showed no

107

evidence of erosions. Patients with chronic arthritis retained very high antibody titres to Chikungunya. None of these patients had positive rheumatoid factor titres[27].

There are reports of a destructive, erosive arthritis developing following Chikungunya infection[29,30]. The association is documented poorly as yet but potentially is very important in rheumatological research. This is the only virus that is implicated in the pathogenesis of destructive, erosive joint disease in man. This form of arthritis may be studied as a human model of chronic destructive joint disease.

It appears that there is a spectrum of response to infection with these arboviruses. The majority recover over a period of weeks or months, but others suffer a greater or lesser degree of residual joint symptoms which may persist for many years and may result in joint erosion. At present, there are no prediction factors for this sub-population. One study suggested that an association exists between possession of the HLA-B27 antigen and susceptibility to the chronic form of Chikungunya arthritis[7]. Of 5 patients with chronic arthritis following an isolated outbreak, 4 were found to be positive for the HLA-B27 antigen. This association has not been found by other workers, including our own unpublished study. No other genetic susceptibility factor has been suggested.

Studies of the chronic form of arbovirus arthritis are hampered by logistical problems. Most cases of arbovirus arthritis occur during epidemics, usually in areas with poor medical facilities. The early cases in such an epidemic are diagnosed serologically. Once the epidemic is established, diagnosis is made on clinical grounds. Hence, very few of the occasional cases which go on to be chronic have been diagnosed serologically in the acute phase. Unless rising viral antibody titres have been demonstrated between acute and convalescent sera, the disease cannot be attributed to the arbovirus because high viral titres are known to persist for many years in some patients.

DIAGNOSIS AND TREATMENT

Definitive diagnosis of arbovirus infection can only be made by isolation of the virus or by serological testing of acute and convalescent sera from an infected patient. Virus isolation from serum is difficult and only possible in the first 2–4 days after appearance of symptoms. Virus isolation from other fluids and tissues has not been reported.

Arboviruses are classified into genera and species according to the results of three types of immunological reactions: complement fixation, neutralization and haemagglutination-inhibition. These reactions are used commonly in the diagnosis of arbivorus infection.

A fourfold rise in antibody titres to a specific virus between acute and convalescent sera indicates recent infection by that virus or a closely related virus.

There is a considerable degree of antigenic overlap demonstrated by antibody cross-reactions amongst many groups of arboviruses and this is the basis of their classification. This phenomenon may represent the sharing of epitopes amongst groups of arboviruses. The overlap was first described after studies on West Nile virus[31], but almost all arboviruses have now been shown to have some antigenic inter-relationships. Diagnosis of infection by one of the alphaviruses described above is usually made by haemagglutination-inhibition testing. An alphavirus will not cross-react with arboviruses of other genera. They will cross-react with other alphaviruses in these reactions but to a lesser degree than with homologous antigen. With other genera, the interrelationships are more complicated and require more comprehensive tests. Similar tests with flaviviruses showed that immune sera raised against a specific virus produced higher haemagglutination-inhibition titres to heterologous antigen from some other flaviviruses[32].

As described previously, diagnosis during an epidemic is usually on clinical grounds. A high index of suspicion is essential in areas where the viruses are endemic.

There are other less specific indicators of arbovirus infection. In the acute phase of the infection, the erythrocyte sedimentation rate is usually raised. Serum acute-phase protein concentrations show a non-specific rise. A leukopaenia with a relative lymphocytosis is usually present. Studies with serum complement vary between arboviruses. Patients with Ross river virus arthritis exhibit no depletion of serum complement and the virus does not activate either the classical or alternative pathway *in vitro* in the absence of the virus-specific antibody[24]. Conversely, Sindbis has been shown to activate both the classical and the alternative pathways[33].

109

Treatment of arbovirus arthritis is unsatisfactory. In the acute phase, pain may be severe, particularly in Chikungunya arthritis. Non-steroidal anti-inflammatory agents, the first-line treatment in other forms of inflammatory arthritis, are ineffective[4]. Opiate analgesics are effective and may be indicated.

No controlled trials of therapy for the chronic form of arbovirus arthritis have been published. Anecdotal evidence and one uncontrolled pilot study suggest that antimalarial drugs may be of value in these patients. In this study[29], chloroquine, in high doses similar to those used for rheumatoid arthritis, was given to 6 patients with chronic Chikungunya arthritis for 3 months. Of these patients, 3 had significantly reduced joint tenderness (measured by the Ritchie articular index), 2 had slight improvement and 1 patient did not improve. Clearly, a larger study is required to confirm these findings. No trials of the other second-line drugs used in rheumatoid arthritis as therapy for chronic arbovirus arthritis had been published.

Prevention of these infections is desirable due to the inadequacy of treatment, severity of the disease in some individuals and the increased number of non-immune tourists visiting areas where these viruses are endemic. Vaccines for other togaviruses, such as rubella and yellow fever, are in widespread use but no vaccines are available commercially for alphaviruses. Several groups have attempted to produce such a vaccine. A vaccine to Chikungunya has been produced[34], and has been shown to be effective against African and Asian strains of the virus.

Of the other measures for prevention of arbovirus infection, vector control is the most promising. An alternative is control of vertebrate amplifier hosts but much more is known of identity and ecology of the vectors than of the hosts.

THE IMPORTANCE OF ARBOVIRUSES

Arboviruses are found all over the world in all climates. In recent years, arboviruses have been discovered even in Northern Europe and the UK. Their spread is limited by the ecology of their hosts and vectors. With the increase in tourism and travel to previously inaccessible parts of the world, it is possible that visitors to areas where arboviruses are endemic may become infected by the virus and return home before symptoms have developed. It is conceivable that such a visitor could return home whilst still in the viraemic phase and infect any suitable local vectors. Hence, a knowledge of arboviruses and the clinical syndromes with which they are associated is a relevant asset to all rheumatologists.

Of greater importance is the enormous worldwide morbidity associated with alphavirus infection. The epidemics of alphavirus infection are amongst the greatest ever recorded. The epidemic of O'nyong nyong in 1959 was reported to affect several million people. The number of cases of endemic alphavirus infection is still increasing, although this may be due, at least in part, to improvement in diagnosis due to increased awareness of these conditions.

Chikungunya arthritis presents an exciting opportunity for research workers as a means of studying the pathogenesis of chronic polyarthritis in man. An important aetiological factor is known. This gives the rheumatologist an opportunity to study the pathogenesis of the condition at an earlier stage than can be achieved by studying other forms of chronic joint disease, such as rheumatoid arthritis. An animal model of Chikungunya arthritis is under development for this purpose. Studies of the virus at the molecular level may also yield information concerning the induction and maintenance of chronic polyarthritis in man.

REFERENCES

1. Theiler, M. and Downs, W. G. (1973). *The Arthropod-Borne Viruses of Vertebrates*, p. 137. (New Haven and London: Yale University Press)
2. Pavri, K. M. (1964). Presence of Chikungunya antibodies in human sera collected from Calcutta and Mashedpur before 1963. *Ind. J. Med. Res.*, **54**, 698–702
3. Halstead, S. and O'Rourke, E. J. (1973). Dengue virus and mononuclear phagocytes. Infection enhancement by non-neutralising antibody. *J. Exp. Med.*, **146**, 210–217
4. Robinson, M. C. (1955). An epidemic of virus disease in Southern Province, Tanganyika Territory in 1952–1953. Clinical features. *Trans. R. Soc. Trop. Med. Hyg.*, **49**, 28–32
5. Carey, D. E. (1971). Chikungunya and Dengue: a case of mistaken identity. *J. Hist. Med.*, **26**, 243–262
6. McIntosh, B. M. (1970). Antibody against chikungunya virus in wild primates in Southern Africa. *S. Afr. J. Med. Sci.*, **35**, 65–74
7. McIntosh, B. M., Paterson, H. E., Donaldson, J. M. and de Sousa, J. (1963).

Chikungunya virus: Viral susceptibility and transmission studies with some vertebrates and mosquitos. *S. Afr. J. Med. Sci.*, **28**, 45–52

8. McIntosh, B. M. and Jupp, P. G. (1970). Attempts to transmit chikungunya virus with six species of mosquito. *J. Med. Entomol.*, **3**, 615–618

9. Fourie, F. D. and Morrison, J. G. L. (1979). Rheumatoid arthritis syndrome after Chikungunya fever. *S. Afr. Med. J.*, **56**, 130–132

10. Kennedy, A. C., Fleming, J. and Solomon, L. (1980). Chikungunya viral arthropathy: a clinical description. *J. Rheumatol.*, **7**, 231–236

11. De Ranitz, C. M., Myers, R. M., Varkey, M. J., Isaac, Z. H. and Carey, D. E. (1965). Clinical expression of Chikungunya in Vellore gained from studies of adult patients. *Ind. J. Med. Res.*, **53**, 707–714

12. Taylor, R. M., Hurlbut, H. S., Work, T. H., Kingston, J. R. and Frothingham, T. E. (1955). Sindbis virus: a newly recognised arthropod-transmitted virus. *Am. J. Trop. Med. Hyg.*, **4**, 844–862

13. McIntosh, B. M., McGillivray, G. M., Dickenson, D. B. and Taljaard, J. J. (1968). Ecological studies on Sindbis and West Nile viruses in South Africa. IV. Infection in a wild avian population. *S. Afr. J. Med. Sci.*, **33**, 105–112

14. Findlay, G. H. and Whiting, D. A. (1968). Arbovirus exanthem from Sindbis and West Nile viruses. *Br. J. Dermatol.*, **80**, 67–74

15. McIntosh, B. M., McGillivray, G. M. Dickenson, D. B. and Malherbe, H. (1964). Illness caused by Sindbis and West Nile viruses in South Africa. *S. Afr. Med. J.*, **38**, 291–294

16. Haddow, A. J., Davies, C. W. and Walker, A. J. (1960). O'nyong nyong fever: an epidemic virus disease in East Africa. 1. Introduction. *Trans. R. Soc. Trop. Med. Hyg.*, **54**, 517–522

17. Shore, H. (1961). O'nyong nyong fever. Some clinical and epidemiological observations. *Trans. R. Soc. Trop. Med. Hyg.*, **55**, 361–373

18. Filipe, A. R. and Pinto, M. R. (1973). Arbovirus studies in Luanda, Angola. *Bull. WHO 1973*, **49**, 37–40

19. Nimmo, J. R. (1928). An unusual epidemic. *Med. J. Aust.*, **1**, 549–550

20. Doherty, R. L., Gorman, B. M., Whitehead, R. H. and Carley, J. G. (1964). Studies of epidemic polyarthritis: The significance of three Group A arboviruses isolated frm mosquitos in Queensland. *Aust. Ann. Med.*, **13**, 322

21. Doherty, R. L., Carley, J. G. and Best, J. C. (1972). Isolation of Ross river virus from man. *Med. J. Aust.*, **1**, 1083–1084

22. Aaskov, J. G., Nair, K., Lawrence, G. W., Dalglish, D. A. and Tucker, M. M. (1981). Evidence for transplacental transmission of Ross River virus in humans. *Med. J. Aust.*, **2**, 20–21

23. Fraser, J. R. E. and Cunningham, A. L. (1980). Incubation time of epidemic polyarthritis. *Med. J. Aust.*, **1**, 550–551

24. Aaskov, J. G., Hadding, U. and Bitter-Suermann, D. (1985). Interaction of Ross River virus with the complement system. *J. Gen. Virol.*, **66**, 121–129

25. Mudge, P. R. (1977). A survey of epidemic polyarthritis in the Riverland area, 1976, *Med. J. Aust.*, **1**, 649–651

26. Anderson, C. R., Downs, W. G., Wattlley, G. H., Ahin, N. W. and Reese, A. A. (1957). Mayaro virus: a new human disease agent. *Am. J. Trop. Med. Hyg.*, **6**, 1012

27. Pinheiro, F. P., Freitas, R. B., da Rosa, J. F. T., Gabby, Y. B., Mello, W. A. and LeDuc, J. W. (1981). An outbreak of Mayaro virus disease in Belterra, Brazil. *Am. J. Trop. Med. Hyg.*, **30**, 674–81

28. Doherty, R. L., Barret, E. J., Gorman, B. M. and Whitehead, R. H. (1971). Epidemic polyarthritis in Eastern Australia, 1959–1970. *Med. J. Aust.,* **1,** 5–7
29. Brighton, S. W. (1983). Third World Rheumatology. In Dick, W. C. and Moll, J. M. H. (eds.) *Recent Advances in Rheumatology 3.,* pp. 97–115. (Edinburgh: Churchill-Livinstone).
30. Brighton, S. W. and Simson, I. W. (1984). A destructive arthropathy following Chikungunya virus arthritis – a possible association. *Clin. Rheum.,* **3,** 253–258
31. Smithburn, K. C. and Jacobs, H. R. (1942). Neutralisation against neurotropic viruses with sera collected in Central Africa. *J. Immunol.,* **44,** 9–23
32. Casals, J. and Brown, L. V. (1954). Haemagglutination with arthropod-borne viruses. *J. Exp. Med.,* **99,** 429–449
33. Hirsch, R. L., Winklestein, J. A. and Griffin, D. E. (1980). Role of complement in viral infection III. Activation of the classical and alternative complement pathways by Sindbis virus. *J. Immunol.,* **124,** 2507–2510
34. Harrison, V. R., Eckels, H., Bartelloni, P. J. and Hampton, C. (1971). Production and evaluation of a formation killed Chikungunya vaccine. *J. Immunol.,* **107,** 643–647

7

MANAGEMENT OF THE SEPTIC JOINT

D. J. WALKER

Septic arthritis remains one of the few true emergencies in rheumatology. The rate at which permanent damage to the structure of the joint occurs demands immediate action on suspicion of sepsis. It is better to treat many cases of gout with antibiotics than to not treat one septic joint.

INITIAL MANAGEMENT

The red hot joint requires aspiration as is discussed elsewhere in this book. It is very important that this should be done prior to treatment with antibiotics. Some joints are easily palpated and aspirated but others, such as the hip and sacroiliac joints, are not. The presence of an effusion in such joints can frequently be confirmed by ultrasound[1]. Aspiration should then be performed by an experienced person using either X-ray or ultrasound to confirm that the joint has been penetrated. A dry tap is not significant unless this has been done. It is not possible to confirm or exclude a diagnosis of infection merely on the basis of inspection or white cell count of the fluid aspirated[2]. If the fluid may be infected, the patient should be treated as though it is, pending the results of culture. Part of the fluid should be microscoped immediately with a Gram stain as this may give an early indication of the likely organism. Inspection of the fluid with a polarizing light microscope is usual because crystal-induced arthritis is the other common cause of a red hot joint. It should be remembered that the presence of crystals in the fluid does not in any way exclude infection. In patients with crystals deposited in their joints, any cause for a joint effusion will show some crystals in the fluid.

Prior to commencing antibiotics, other potentially informative tests should be performed. A portal of entry for the bacteria into the body, such as a boil, should be sought and, if found, swabbed. Blood should be taken for culture as this is occasionally the only source from which the organism is isolated. An erythrocyte sedimentation rate (ESR) should be measured, not to assist in diagnosis, but to provide a way of following the progress of the disease. Radiographs of the affected joint are important and the radiological changes in septic arthritis are reviewed by Resnick[3]. X-rays will show up any pre-existing joint problems or nearby osteomyelitis, which may cause joint effusion, either sterile or septic[4]. These X-rays will act as a base line for progression of the disease.

The use of radioisotope scanning techniques, such as labelling leukocytes with gallium or indium, has only a small part to play in defining septic arthritis[5]. While these scans can give results suggestive of the presence of localized infection, this is only useful if performed in a patient with good evidence of sepsis, but at an unknown site. This site may be a joint.

Computerized tomography (CT) and nuclear magnetic resonance (NMR) are also only occasionally useful. Both are good for defining the extent of the infection, particularly in the surrounding bone[6] and NMR may be better than CT[7].

Some general principles of management apply to any patient with septic arthritis. The patient should be admitted to hospital for bed rest and observation. The affected joint should be splinted, if accessible, to ensure maximum rest. Temperature should be taken four-hourly. Unaffected limbs should receive maintenance physiotherapy, particularly in the presence of other, pre-existing, arthritis.

Antibiotics should be started prior to culture results being available. The choice of antibiotic and route of administration may vary according to local considerations and the co-operation of a microbiologist is important. In an adult patient who was previously fit and well, the most likely causative organism is a staphylococcus. Treatment with parenteral flucloxacillin, 500 mg four times daily, is therefore the initial treatment. In other circumstances, different antibiotics may be preferable. The experience of culturing synovial fluid samples from RA patients at the Freeman Road Hospital is that only 50% isolate staphylococci and the rest other organisms, particularly *Escherichia coli*. For this reason, it is now our policy to commence treatment with more broad spectrum antibiotics. Currently, we use cefuroxime, 750 mg intravenously, eight-hourly pending the results of culture and sensitivity. It may be that the even more powerful broad spectrum antibiotics which are becoming available will find a place in treating this sort of patient[8]. In babies under the age of two years, *Haemophilus influenzae* is the most usual cause of septic arthritis[9] and hence the choice of antibiotic should reflect this. In drug addicts, pseudomonas and klebsiella are common pathogens and the spine and sacroiliac joints are frequently involved[10]. The gonococcus frequently causes polyarticular sepsis[9] and sexually active females should have high vaginal swabs taken.

The presence of polyarthritis, such as rheumatoid arthritis, will influence management. In such patients, sepsis should be considered if one joint becomes inflamed out of proportion to the rest of the arthritis. The choice of antibiotic may be altered as discussed above. The need to keep the patient's other limbs active may dictate earlier mobilization.

Drug therapy for pre-existing arthritis may influence the presentation and progress of the disease. Corticosteroids will not only increase the risk of sepsis but they may also mask the symptoms and delay presentation. It is, however, rarely possible to stop such steroid therapy; in fact, it is usually necessary to increase the steroids during the infection to allow for adrenal supression. Non-steroidal anti-inflammatory drugs may produce similar problems but to a lesser degree. Cases of septic arthritis occasionally show dramatic symptomatic response to NSAIDs, causing delay in specific therapy and probably a worse outcome. It is well known that NSAIDs, such as indomethacin, will severely inhibit the function of macrophages *in vitro*[11]. As macrophage function is important in clearing infection, there is some argument as to whether NSAID therapy should be stopped during septic arthritis.

FURTHER MANAGEMENT

Once the results of culture and sensitivity are available, the antibiotic should be changed accordingly, with the advice of a microbiologist. If no organism is isolated from any of the cultures and the joint is still thought to be infected, broad spectrum antibiotics should be continued. It is our policy to convert to oral cephalexin, 500 mg, eight-hourly, after one week. Response then has to be judged clinically and with the help of the ESR.

Adequate drainage of the affected joint is essential to minimize joint damage. Should effusion recur in the affected joint, it must be drained. It is usually possible to keep a joint adequately drained by repeated needle aspiration, but, if this proves difficult, the help of an orthopaedic surgeon will be invaluable. The surgeon will be able to perform an arthrotomy and place drains, allowing irrigation with antiseptics, such as Noxyflex. Arthroscopy, as a method of drainage, may be a less invasive way of surgically draining a septic joint[12].

The patient should be kept in bed until the joint is clinically quiet. ESR will tend to follow the clinical progress but with a delay of a week or two. Radiographs should be repeated after one week but may be expected to deteriorate for several weeks after active infection has been eradicated.

The duration of antibiotic therapy should be between six weeks and three months. In circumstances where the infection proves difficult to eradicate, antibiotics may need to be continued indefinitely.

LATE MANAGEMENT

Over the weeks following treatment, the extent of the permanent damage to the joint will become apparent. This will be judged both clinically and radiologically. Symptoms should be treated on their merit as for degenerative arthritis. Should the pain and disability be severe enough, orthopaedic opinion about arthroplasty should be sought. Such opinion may vary with different surgeons. Some surgeons will not consider arthroplasty following sepsis but will favour arthrodesis. Others will replace the joint once infection is eradicated.

INFECTION IN THE PRESENCE OF AN ARTIFICIAL JOINT

Infection is a rare, but disastrous, complication of arthroplasty, either at the time of operation or subsequently, and prophylactic antibiotics should be taken for potentially bacteraemic procedures. Infection usually presents with pain and swelling of the affected joint and loosening of the prosthesis. Systemic signs of infection are usually present. The first investigation in this situation should be a radiograph[13] and this is most likely to show a lucent zone around the prosthesis, or the cement, of greater than 2 mm. On suspicion of infection, orthopaedic help should be sought immediately. Eradication of the infection without removal of the artificial joint is rare[14]. It is, however, sometimes possible to suppress infection with long-term antibiotics and this may be preferable to removing the joint. Revision of an infected arthroplasty is possible but orthopaedic opinion is again divided. Some encouraging results have been achieved using antibiotic-impregnated cement[15]. An alternative is to remove the infected joint, keep the patient in traction for several weeks until the infection is eradicated and then replace the joint. Again, this is not straight-forward as the complete removal of the cement is difficult. In the case of the hip joint of an elderly person, a Girdlestone's procedure may be satisfactory.

REFERENCES

1. Lopez, M. *et al.* (1985). Ultrasonography and C.T. in the assessment of septic arthritis of the hip in adults. *J. Can. Assoc. Radiol.*, **36**, 322–324
2. Platt, P. N. (1983). Examination of synovial fluid. *Clin. Rheum. Dis.*, **9**, 51–68
3. Resnick, D. (1982). Infectious arthritis. *Semin. Roentgenol.*, **137**, 721–723
4. Platt, P. N. and Griffiths, I. D. (1984). Pyogenic osteomyelitis presenting as an acute sterile arthropathy. *Ann. Rheum. Dis.*, **43**, 607–609
5. McAfee, J. G. and Samin, A. (1985). In-111 labeled leucocytes: a review of problems in image interpretation. *Radiology*, **155**, 221–229
6. Wing, V. W., Jeffrey, R. B., Federle, M. P., Helms, C. A. and Trafton, P. (1985). Chronic osteomyelitis examined by C.T. *Radiology*, **154**, 171–174
7. Fletcher, B. D., Scoles, P. V. and Nelson, A. D. (1984). Osteomyelitis in children: detection by magnetic resonance imaging. *Radiology*, **150**, 57–60
8. Giamarellou, H. (1987). Newer pathogens and clinical experience of newer anti-microbials in the adult. *Proc. Eur. Cong. Rheumatol.*, Suppl. Athens 1987, 30–33
9. Fink, C. W. and Nelson, J. D. (1986). Septic arthritis and osteomyelitis in children. *Clin. Rheum. Dis.*, **12**, 423–435

10. Roca, R. P. and Yoshikawa, T. T. (1979). Primary skeletal infections in heroin users. *Clin. Orthop. Relat. Res.*, **144,** 238–248
11. Famaey, J-P., Brookes, P. M. and Dick, W. C. (1975). Biological effects of non-steroidal anti-inflammatory drugs. *Semin. Arthritis Rheum.*, **5,** 63–81
12. Jackson, R. W. (1985). The septic knee: arthroscopic treatment. *Arthroscopy,* **1** (3), 194–197
13. Brause, B. D. (1986) Infections associated with prosthetic joints. *Clin. Rheum. Dis.*, **12,** 523–536
14. Fitzgerald, R. H., Nolan, D. R. and Ilstrup, D. M. (1977). Deep wound sepsis following total hip arthroplasty. *J. Bone Jt. Surg.*, **59a,** 847–855
15. Carlsson, A. S., Josefsson, G. and Lindberg, L. (1978). Revision with gentamycin-impregnated cement for deep infections in total hip arthroplasties. *J. Bone Jt. Surg.*, **60a,** 1059–1064

8

INTERLEUKIN 1 AND TUMOUR NECROSIS FACTOR IN THE PATHOGENESIS OF SEPTIC ARTHRITIS

F. S. DI GIOVINE, J. A. SYMONS and G. W. DUFF

Septic arthritis is a medical emergency requiring early diagnosis and effective antimicrobial treatment. Though the great majority of cases have a satisfactory outcome, one of the most striking features is the rapid destruction of cartilage and bone tissue that can occur, frequently leading to permanent joint damage.

The cellular and molecular mechanisms of tissue destruction during inflammation and infection are incompletely understood, but significant progress has been made recently and it seems certain that the induction of cytokines will be established as an important event in the pathogenesis.

Cytokines are inducible proteins with receptor-mediated effects on many different target cells. Cells of macrophage lineage, lymphocytes, endothelial and other mesenchymal cells have the potential to produce cytokines after appropriate stimulation. In articular pathology, the cytokines that have received most attention so far have been the interleukins and cytotoxins[1,2]. In particular, interleukin 1 α and β and tumour necrosis factor α have powerful effects on the metabolism of bone[3,4] and cartilage tissues[5,6]. These proteins[7,8] have already been implicated in the pathogenesis of several rheumatic diseases, including rheumatoid arthritis, reactive arthritis, crystal-associated arthritis and septic arthritis.

INTERLEUKIN 1

Interleukin 1 peptides are produced by 2 distinct genes (IL1 α and β)[9]. The genes are structurally similar, with 7 exons, 6 introns and related 3′ untranslated regions in their mRNA[10,11]. In both cases, the primary translation product is a propeptide of approximately 31 kDa which is then processed to produce mature peptides of 17 kDa[9]. Though the peptides share only 26% homology in amino acid sequence they compete equally for binding to a single class of receptor on target tissue[12,13]. Consequently, and especially *in vitro*, their biological activities are very similar[14]. However, there are important differences between the two proteins, and, while neither carries a classical hydrophobic leader sequence typical of secretory proteins, IL1 β achieves about 60% extracellular translocation while IL1 α remains more than 90% cell associated[15].

TABLE 8.1   Molecular characteristics of human IL1 and TNF

	IL1 α	IL1 β	TNF α
Gene location	chromosome 2	unpublished	chromosome 6 (in MHC)
mRNA	2.2 kb	1.6 kb	1.6/1.8 kb
Propeptide	271aa 30.6 kDa	269aa 30.7 kDa	233aa
Glycosylation	no	one potential site	no
Leader sequence	no	no	76aa
Mature peptide	159aa 17.5 kDa pI 5	153aa 17.3 kDa pI 7	157aa 17.4 kDa
Native molecule	monomer or non-covalent polymer	monomer or non-covalent polymer	non-covalent polymers
Receptor	80 kDa also IL1 β	80 kDa also IL1 α	70 kDa/138 kDa also TNF β

The IL1 receptor has been characterized and cloned[16]. It is a peptide of approximately 80 kDa which retains affinity for IL1 even when in solution. Table 8.1 summarizes some of the molecular and biochemical properties of IL1 α and β.

IL1 bioactivities are extremely wide ranging and biological effects can be seen with concentrations as low as 10^{-15} mol L^{-1}. Of the many effects attributed to IL1, those relevant to joint destruction include

TABLE 8.2   Some biological effects of IL1 *in vitro*

IMMUNE SYSTEM	MUSCULOSKELETAL TISSUE
T-cells	**Bone**
Comitogenic with antigen	Resorption (organ culture)
IL2 induction	Osteoclast activation
IL2R expression	Osteoblast mitogenesis
IL4 production	
IFN γ induction	**Cartilage**
IL3 induction	Resorption (organ culture)
c-fos/c-myc induction	
Chemotaxis	**Chondrocytes**
	Release of collagenase
B-cells	Release of plasminogen activator
BCGF activity (proliferation) – cofactor?	Release of neutral proteases
BCDF activity (ab production) – cofactor?	Activation of PLA_2
	Decreased collagen synthesis
Monocytes	Decreased proteoglycan synthesis
Chemotaxis	
Cytotoxicity enhancement	**Fibroblasts**
PGE_2 synthesis	Proliferation
IL1 autoinduction	PGE_2 production
	Collagenase induction
NK cells	Cytokine production
Enhancement in NK activity (with IL2?)	Increased collagen synthesis
	Decreased collagen synthesis (via PGE?)
Basophils	
Degranulation, histamine release	**Synoviocytes**
	PGE_2 production
Eosinophils	Collagenase induction
Degranulation	
	VASCULAR TISSUES
Fibroblasts	**Endothelial cells**
Induction of:	Proliferation
IFN β 2/IL6	Thromboxane production
GM-CSF	PGI_2 production
PGE_2 and proteases	Procoagulant activity
	PGE_2 production
Endothelial cells	Increased adhesiveness
Induction of:	Cytokine production
GM-CSF	
M-CSF	**Vascular smooth muscle**
IL1	IL1 autoinduction
ICAM 1 protein	

the properties of inducing chondrocytes to resorb proteoglycan matrix in cartilage[17] – an activity of IL1 previously described as 'catabolin'; the activation of osteoclasts and the induction of bone resorption[18]; and the stimulation of synovial cells to produce proteinolytic enzymes such as collagenase, and proinflammatory mediators including prostaglandin E2[19].

Direct evidence of the arthritogenic properties of IL1 has now been obtained in animal experiments[20,21] where the injection of recombinant or purified IL1 directly into joints was followed by synovial fluid leukocytosis, proteoglycan breakdown and lymphocyte infiltration. It is, therefore, clear that IL1 has the potential to mediate joint destruction. Some relevant biological activities of interleukin 1 α and β are listed in Tables 8.2 and 8.3.

TABLE 8.3   Some biological activities of IL1 *in vivo*

Hypotension
Fever
Slow-wave sleep
Anorexia, weight loss
Neutrophilia
Acute-phase proteins (SAA, SAP, fibrinogen, CRP, α-1 AT, C3)
Plasma metal levels
   hypozincaemia
   hypoferraemia
   hypercupraemia
Increased hormone levels
   corticosterone, ACTH, insulin, glucagon
Bone marrow cell-cycling
Induction of circulating CSFs
Adjuvant effect
Decreased cytochrome P450 enzyme activity
Neutrophil accumulation in joints
Cartilage proteoglycan breakdown
Enhanced resistance to bacterial infection

TUMOUR NECROSIS FACTOR α

This cytokine was previously identified by its cytotoxicity for certain tumour cell lines and also its role in inducing cachexia in infected animals[22]. It is an inducible, classical secretory protein with a hydrophobic leader sequence, and 95% of newly synthesized tumour necrosis factor α is released extracellularly within 20 hours[15]. Its biological effects are very similar to those of interleukin 1 though it is the product of a different gene and acts via a distinct cell surface receptor (see Table 8.1). Of relevance to inflammatory arthritis and joint tissue destruction, it shares with IL1 the ability to induce cartilage[6] and bone[4] resorption and also activates synovial cells for the production of mediators of tissue damage such as collagenase[23].

Tumour necrosis factor (TNF) α and both IL1 α and β (Table 8.2) have profound effects on the immune system through the stimulation of lymphocyte growth factors and their receptors[24,25]. In particular, the induction of interleukin 2 and its receptor by interleukin 1 have been well documented[25,26]. Another cytokine[27] induced by IL1 and TNF is interleukin 6 which is now regarded as a major mediator of the acute phase response with regulatory activities on the expression of acute phase protein genes, major histocompatibility complex genes and the pro-opiomelanocortin gene from which endocrine peptides, such as adrenocorticotrophin and α melanocyte stimulating hormone, are processed. Thus, many biological effects of IL1 and TNF may be indirect and mediated by the induction of other cytokines in a classical biological amplification cascade.

THE INDUCTION OF IL1 AND TNF

In most studies, it has been concluded that the genes encoding IL1 α and β and TNF α are not constitutively expressed. Gene expression occurs after cellular activation with extrinsic stimuli. In human blood monocytes, resting cells do not contain detectable mRNA for IL1 α or β nor for TNF α. Specific mRNA accumulates in the cell within minutes of cell activation and the kinetics of accumulation of mRNA and protein are broadly parallel, suggesting that a major level of control occurs at the stage of gene transcription[9,15]. Stimuli for gene transcription are generated during immune responses and include a range of lymphocyte secretory proteins (lymphokines) as well as immune complexes and possibly cellular aggregation, suggesting that signals transduced through lymphokine receptors, Fc and/or complement receptors and adhesion molecules can all regulate expression of IL1 and TNF genes. Thus, immunogenic microbial pathogens will stimulate IL1 and TNF production from antigen presenting cells indirectly by lymphocyte-mediated mechanisms, but it has also been known for many years that most microbial agents can stimulate cytokine production from monocytes directly by an action on the monocyte membrane[28].

Perhaps the best example of a microbial product capable of direct activation of monocyte production of IL1 and TNF is the endotoxin (lipopolysaccharide, LPS) component of the cell walls of Gram-negative organisms. Bacterial LPS, and in particular the lipid A moiety of this macromolecule, has long been used in experimental study of cytokine induction from macrophages. Typical dose-dependent induction of IL1 from normal human blood monocytes stimulated by bacterial LPS is shown in Figure 8.1. Biologically detectable IL1 activity is induced by LPS concentrations as low as $20\,\mathrm{pg\,ml}^{-1}$ and below if cells are primed by γ-interferon. Clearly, infection with a Gram-negative organism will cause direct activation of resident and recruited macrophages and lead to the production of IL1 and TNF. LPS is, of course, not the only microbial product capable of direct stimulation of cytokine gene expression, and Gram-positive bacteria, viruses and yeasts are all potent stimuli of IL1 and TNF production. Table 8.4 lists some reported microbial stimuli of IL1 production and release. An example of TNF α induction in human monocytes stimulated with heat-killed staphylococci is shown in Figure 8.2. This is a direct effect and is independent of phagocytosis.

CLINICAL MEASUREMENT OF CYTOKINES

Historically, most cytokines were recognized first by bioassay. For example, the T-cell activating properties of IL1 were studied as 'lymphocyte activating factor' for many years. This assay measured the comitogenic effect of IL1 on murine thymocytes which had been

126

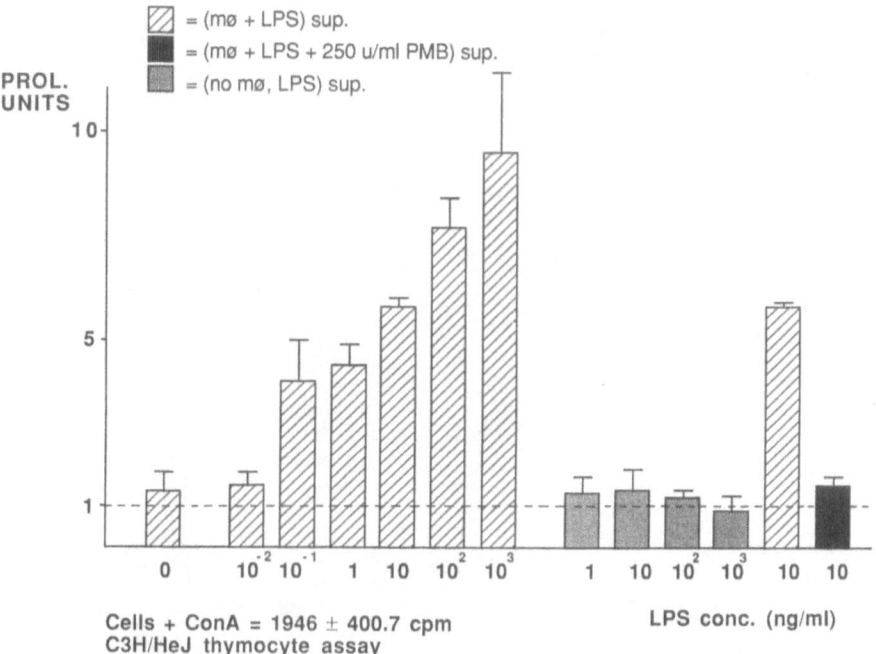

PROL.
UNITS

= (mø + LPS) sup.
= (mø + LPS + 250 u/ml PMB) sup.
= (no mø, LPS) sup.

Cells + ConA = 1946 ± 400.7 cpm
C3H/HeJ thymocyte assay

LPS conc. (ng/ml)

FIGURE 8.1   In this experiment, human blood monocytes from a healthy donor were separated by density centrifugation and adherence and cultured at 10^6/ml. *E. coli* LPS, at the concentrations indicated, was added to the culture and 20-hour supernatants were tested for IL1 content in the conventional lymphocyte-activating factor assay using thymocytes from an LPS-hyposensitive murine strain. IL1-like activity is indicated in proliferation units on the vertical axis. As indicated in the grey columns, LPS alone in a range of concentrations had no effect on thymocyte proliferation. The hatched columns show IL1-like activity induced in a concentration-dependent manner by LPS and the black column confirmed that IL1 induction was due to LPS since it is neutralized by the antibiotic polymyxin B, which complexes with LPS and neutralizes its biological actions. These results indicate that LPS, at concentrations as low as 10–100 pg/ml, induces IL1 in this system and similar results are obtained with synovial macrophages. TNF production is also stimulated by LPS. It can also be seen that, in the absence of stimulation, the cells do not produce detectable IL1

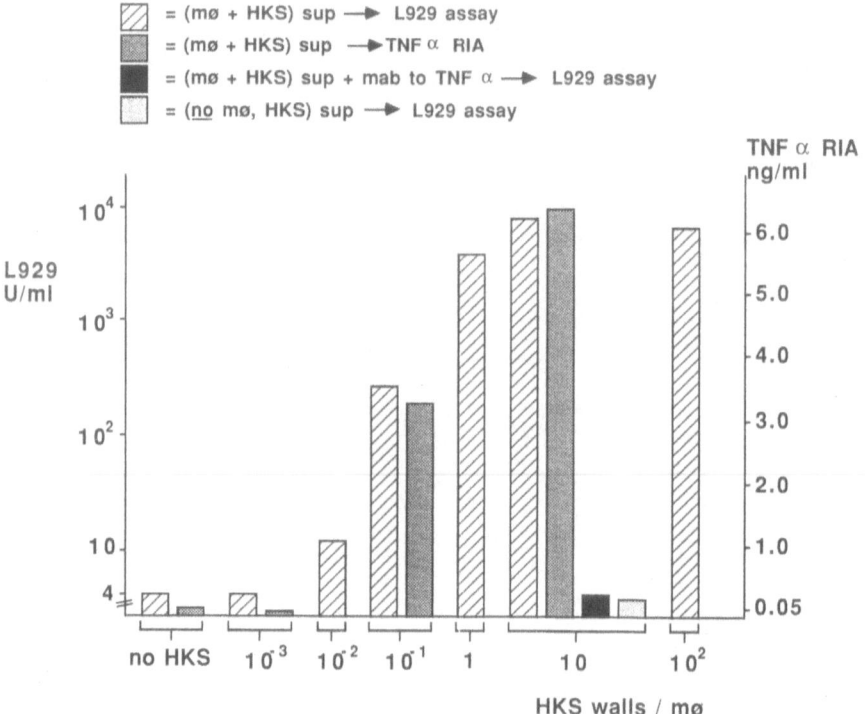

FIGURE 8.2   In this experiment, human blood monocytes from a healthy donor were cultured at 10^6/ml with different concentrations of cell walls of heat-killed staphylococci. Twenty-hour supernatants were tested both for TNF-like biological activity and specific TNF α immunoreactivity in a radioimmunoassay. Biological activity was tested in the conventional cytotoxicity assay using L929 cells (a murine adipocyte/fibroblast cell line). Cells cultured alone produced no significant TNF α but concentration-dependent induction was seen with heat-killed staphylococci. Biological activity and immunoreactivity of TNF α were closely parallel and biological activity was completely neutralized by monoclonal antibody specific for TNF α. Bacterial cell walls alone had no effect in the L929 assay. Heat-killed staphylococci also stimulate IL1 production and similar results to these with blood monocytes can be obtained using synovial adherent cells

suboptimally stimulated with mitogens. Tumour necrosis factor was measured by its cytotoxicity *in vitro* for certain transformed cell lines. Both IL1 and TNF were measured as 'endogenous pyrogen' activity

TABLE 8.4 Direct induction of IL1 by microbial agents

Agent	Target cells
Viruses	
Influenza	Leukocytes
EBV	B-cells
HTLV 1	T-cell lines
Bacteria	
Gram-positive:	
Peptidoglycans	Leukocytes
Muramyl dipeptide	Monocytes
Staphylococcus aureus:	
28 kDa enterotoxin	Leukocytes
12 kDa exotoxin	Leukocytes
Toxic shock exotoxin	Monocytes
Streptococcus:	
Dick's toxin(s)	Leukocytes
Gram-negative:	
Endotoxin (LPS)	Leukocytes
	Monocytes
	B-cells
	Langerhans cells
	Dendritic cells
	NK cells
	Endothelial cells
	Astrocytes
	Mesangial cells
Spirochetae	
Borrelia burgdorferi (Lyme disease)	Monocytes
Fungi	
S. cerevisiae	Leukocytes

in rabbits, and as 'mononuclear cell factor' activity which involved the stimulation of prostaglandins and collagenase from synovial cells. The reliance on bioassays was not compatible with rapid progress in understanding the role of these and similar cytokines *in vivo*. Since many cytokines have similar actions, in most biological assays prob-

129

lems of specificity arise and also, most biological fluids such as plasma, serum and inflammatory exudate, contain agents which interfere with the biological response being measured. However, with the purification, sequencing and subsequent cloning of individual cytokines it became possible to generate monoclonal antibodies or monospecific antisera using recombinant protein as antigen and these developments have enabled specific immunoassay of cytokines, even in biological fluids[7,29,30].

Using immunoassays, IL1 α, IL1 β and TNF α (among other cytokines) have now unequivocally been detected in synovial fluids[7] and other exudates from a number of inflammatory diseases. In septic arthritis, IL1 and TNF have been measured at high concentrations within the active joint on initial presentation and have been shown to fall when inflammation is subsiding following effective antibacterial treatment. An example of this is shown in Table 8.5.

Raised levels of immunoreactive cytokines in synovial fluids from a variety of different rheumatic diseases make it clear that the release of cytokines is not a specific event in the pathogenesis of any particular clinical entity. It seems more likely that cytokine production is a relatively fundamental and early event in the pathogenesis of inflammation. The extent and duration of cytokine release will be influenced by the continuing presence of stimuli such as microbial agents and products of immune responses directed against them or to cross-reactive autoantigens or those revealed by tissue damage. Once produced, the biological effects of IL1 and TNF are likely to be

TABLE 8.5 Immunoassay of cytokines in synovial exudate from septic arthritis (ng/ml)

	IL1 β	IL1 α	TNF α
Day 1	8.1	0.1	1.2
Day 14	4.0	<0.025	0.4

The patient presented with acute monoarthritis. On day 1 staphylococcal colonies were cultured from synovial exudate and antibacterial therapy was given. By day 14 the signs of inflammation in the knee had largely resolved and residual synovial exudate was sterile. Immunoassays for the three cytokines indicated were performed on synovial fluid samples from day 1 and day 14 affected (both positively and negatively) by other cytokines, binding molecules and agents which regulate the expression of their surface receptors on target cells. There is, at present, intense research activity[31,32] aimed at the regulation of cytokine homeostasis and disturbances that may contribute to the pathogenesis of infectious and immune-mediated tissue damage[33].

In summary, IL1 α and β and TNF α have been implicated as mediators of tissue damage in septic arthritis. The evidence for this is:

1. IL1 and TNF unequivocally induce collagenase release from synovial cells, influence proteoglycan and collagen synthesis, induce proteoglycan matrix resorption in cartilage and also stimulate bone resorption (Tables 8.2 and 8.3).

2. Intra-articular injection of IL1 in animals leads to cartilage breakdown and leukocytosis.

3. Human macrophages (including synovial cells) *in vitro* produce IL1 and TNF as a direct response to bacterial products.

4. IL1 α, IL1 β, and TNF are detectable at raised levels by immunoassay in active septic arthritis and levels fall after antibacterial treatment.

Septic arthritis is a good model for tissue destruction in inflammatory joint disease since it has the great advantage of a known aetiological agent. It seems likely that an increased understanding of the role of cytokines and agents that modulate them will lead to new approaches for prevention and possibly reversal of joint damage in many rheumatic diseases.

REFERENCES

1. Powanda, M. C., Oppenheim, J. J., Kluger, M. J. and Dinarello, C. A. (eds.) (1988). *Monokines and Other Non-Lymphocytic Cytokines*, Vol. 8 (New York: Alan R. Liss, Inc.)

2. Bock, J. and Marsh, J. (eds.) (1987). *Tumour Necrosis Factor and Related Cytotoxins*, Ciba Foundation Symposium (Chichester, UK: J. Wiley)

3. Gowen, M., Wood, D. D., Ihrie, E. J., McGuire, M. K. B., Graham, R. and Russel, R. G. G. (1983). An interleukin 1-like factor stimulates bone resorption in vitro. *Nature (London)*, **306**, 378–380

4. Bertolini, D. R., Nedwin, G. E., Bringman, T. S., Smith, D. D. and Mundy, G. R. (1986). Stimulation of bone resorption and inhibition of bone formation in vitro by human tumor necrosis factor. *Nature (London)*, **319**, 516–518
5. Saklatvala, J. (1981). Characterization of catabolin, the major product of synovial tissue that induces resorption of cartilage proteoglycan in vitro. *Biochem. J.*, **199**, 705–714
6. Saklatvala, J. (1986). Tumour necrosis factor alpha stimulates resorption and inhibits synthesis of proteoglycan in cartilage. *Nature (London)*, **322**, 547–549
7. Duff, G. W., Dickens, E., Wood, N., Manson, J., Symons, J., Poole, S. and di Giovine, F. S. (1988). Immunoassay, bioassay and in situ hybridization of mono-kines in human arthritis. In Powanda, M. C., Oppenheim, J. J., Kluger, M. J. and Dinarello, C. A. (eds.) *Monokines and Other Non-Lymphocytic Cytokines*, pp. 387–392. (New York: Alan R. Liss, Inc.)
8. Di Giovine, F. S., Nuki, G. and Duff, G. W. (1988). Tumour necrosis factor in synovial exudates. *Ann. Rheum. Dis.*, **47**, 768–772
9. March, C. J., Mosley, B., Larsen, A., Cerretti, D. P., Braedt, G., Price, V., Gillis, S., Henney, C. S., Kronheimm, S. R., Grabstein, K., Conlon, P. J., Hopp, T. P. and Cosman, D. (1985). Cloning, sequencing and expression of two distinct human interleukin 1 complementary cDNAs. *Nature (London)*, **315**, 641–647
10. Clark, D. B., Collins, K. L., Gandy, M. S., Webb, A. C. and Auron, P. E. (1986). Genomic sequence for human prointerleukin 1 beta – possible evolution from a reverse transcribed prointerleukin 1 alpha gene. *Nucleic Acids Res.*, **14**, 7897–7914
11. Furutani, Y., Notake, M., Fukui, T., Ohue, M., Nomura, H., Yamada, M. and Nakamura, S. (1986). Complete nucleotide sequence of the gene for human interleukin 1 alpha. *Nucleic Acids Res.*, **14**, 3167–3179
12. Dower, S. K., Kronheim, S. R., March, C. J., Conlon, P. J., Hopp, T. D., Gillis, S. and Urdal, D. (1985). Detection and characterization of high affinity plasma membrane receptors for human interleukin 1. *J. Exp. Med.*, **162**, 501–515
13. Bird, T. A. and Saklatvala, J. (1986). Identification of a common class of high affinity receptors for both types of porcine interleukin 1 on connective tissue cells. *Nature (London)*, **324**, 263–266
14. Dinarello, C. A. (1986). Interleukin 1: aminoacid sequences, multiple biological activities and comparison with tumor necrosis factor (cachectin). *Year Immunol.*, **2**, 68–89
15. Di Giovine, F. S., Symons, J. A. and Duff, G. W. (1988). Kinetics of cytokine mRNA and protein accumulation in activated monocytes. (In press)
16. Sims, J. E., March, C. J., Cosman, D., Widmer, M. B., Robson MacDonald, H., McMahan, C. J., Grubin, C. E., Wignall, J. M., Jackson, J. L., Call, S. D., Friend, D., Alpert, A. R., Gillis, S., Urdal, D. L. and Dower, S. K. (1988). cDNA expression and cloning of the IL1 receptor, a member of the immunoglobulin superfamily. *Science*, **241**, 585–589
17. Saklatvala, J., Sarsfield, S. J. and Townsend, Y. (1985). Pig interleukin 1. Puri-fication of two immunologically different leukocyte proteins that cause cartilage resorption, lymphocyte activation, and fever. *J. Exp. Med.*, **162**, 1208–1222
18. Gowen, M., Wood, D. D., Ihrie, E. J., Meats, J. E. and Russell, R. G. G. (1984). Stimulation by human interleukin 1 of cartilage breakdown and production of collagenase and proteoglycanase by human chondrocytes but not by human osteoblasts in vitro. *Biochim. Biophys. Acta.*, **797**, 186–193

19. Dayer, J. M., Krane, S. M., Russell, R. G. G. and Robinson, D. R. (1976). Production of collagenase and prostaglandins by isolated adherent rheumatoid synovial cells. *Proc. Natl. Acad. Sci. USA*, **73**, 945–951

20. Pettipher, E. R., Higgs, G. A. and Henderson, B. (1986). Interleukin 1 induces leukocyte infiltration and cartilage proteoglycan degradation in the synovial joint. *Proc. Natl. Acad. Sci. USA*, **83**, 8749–8753

21. Dingle, J. T., Page, D. P., King, T. B. and Bard, D. R. (1987). In vivo studies of articular tissue damage mediated by catabolin/interleukin 1. *Ann. Rheum. Dis.*, **46**, 527–533

22. Beutler, B. and Cerami, A. (1986). Cachectin and tumour necrosis factor as two sides of the same biological coin. *Nature (London)*, **320**, 584–588

23. Dayer, J. M., Beutler, B. and Cerami, A. (1985). Cachectin/tumor necrosis factor stimulates collagenase and prostaglandin E_2 production by human synovial cells and dermal fibroblasts. *J. Exp. Med.*, **162**, 2163–2168

24. Dinarello, C. A. (1987). The biology of interleukin 1 and comparison to tumour necrosis factor. *Immunol. Lett.*, **16**, 227–232

25. Durum, S. K., Schmidt, J. A. and Oppenheim, J. J. (1985). Interleukin 1: an immunological perspective. *Annu. Rev. Immunol.*, **3**, 263–287

26. Kaye, J., Gillis, S., Mizel, S. B., Shevach, E. M., Malek, T. R., Dinarello, C. A., Lachman, L. B. and Janeway, C. A. (1984). Growth of a cloned helper T-cell line induced by a monoclonal antibody specific for the antigen receptor: interleukin 1 is required for the expression of receptors for interleukin 2. *J. Immunol.*, **133**, 1339–1344

27. Van Damme, J., DeLey, M., Van Snick, J., Dinarello, C. A. and Billiau, A. (1987). The role of interferon beta and the 26 kD protein (interferon beta 2) as mediators of the antiviral effect of interleukin 1 and tumour necrosis factor. *J. Immunol.*, **139**, 1867–1872

28. Atkins, E. (1960). The pathogenesis of fever. *Physiol. Rev.*, **40**, 580–646

29. Eastgate, J. A., Symons, J. A., Wood, N. C., Grinlinton, F. M., di Giovine, F. S. and Duff, G. W. (1988). Correlation of plasma interleukin 1 levels with disease activity in rheumatoid arthritis. *Lancet*, **2**, 706–709

30. Di Giovine, F. S., Meager, A., Leung, H. and Duff, G. W. (1988). Immunoreactive tumour necrosis factor alpha and biological inhibitor(s) in synovial fluids from rheumatic patients. *Int. J. Immunopathol. Pharmacol.*, **1**, 17–26

31. Symons, J. A., Wood, N. C., Di Giovine, F. S. and Duff, G. W. (1988). Soluble IL-2 receptor in rheumatoid arthritis: correlation with disease activity, IL-1, and IL-2 inhibition. *J. Immunol.*, **141**, 2612–2618

32. Manson, J. C., Symons, J. A., di Giovine, F. S., Poole, S. and Duff, G. W. (1988). Autoregulation of interleukin 1 production. *Eur. J. Immunol.* (In press)

33. Wood, N. C., Symons, J. A. and Duff, G. W. (1988). Serum interleukin-2-receptor in rheumatoid arthritis: a prognostic indicator of disease activity? *J. Autoimmun.*, **1**, 353–361

9

ROLE OF POLYMORPHONUCLEAR LEUKOCYTES IN THE PATHOGENESIS OF INFECTIVE ARTHRITIS

I. N. BIRD

INTRODUCTION

Types of arthritis whose onset can be associated with a known infection, diagnosed by the presence of the infective agent or its antigen(s) in the infected joints, are termed infective arthropathies. Infective agents causing such arthropathies are reviewed in the preceding chapters and include bacteria, mycoplasma, fungi and viruses. The arthropathies tend to be acute, with varying patterns of symptoms, and the time taken for resolution is very variable. A major feature of these arthropathies is the increased concentration of polymorphonuclear leukocytes (PMNL) in the synovial fluid.

Normal synovial fluid[1] contains less than 50 white cells/mm^3. In infective arthritis, the white cell count is elevated, the degree of elevation being dependent primarily on the nature of the causative agent; in many forms of infective arthritis, the white cell count can be elevated[1] to greater than 10 000 cells/mm^3. Normally, about 90% of these white cells are PMNL. The cells are engaged in phagocytosis of immune complexes, micro-organisms and cellular debris present in the synovial fluid and surrounding tissue.

Infective arthropathies display, to a greater or lesser extent, the classical signs of acute inflammation, namely redness and swelling with heat, pain and loss of function. At a molecular level, it is more appropriate to envisage inflammation as a collection of distinct mechanisms which defend the body against external injury, each of which have additional functions[2]. Three changes occur in the infected joint:

(1) Changes in vascular calibre and blood flow;
(2) Increased vascular permeability which results in the formation of inflammatory exudate and local oedema;
(3) Escape of leukocytes from the blood into the extravascular tissues[3].

Inflammatory mediators produced by the local tissues and from the activation of systems found in the plasma, such as the kinin, complement and coagulation systems, mediate the extent of the changes seen. In addition, mediators produced by activated PMNL, such as prostaglandins and leukotrienes, contribute to the extent of the inflammation observed.

Since PMNL are the major white blood cell type involved in the acute inflammatory response associated with infective arthritis their role is of great importance. In the course of resolving the infection, PMNL produce large quantities of reactive oxygen species and destructive enzymes. Although the primary function of these products is to ensure that foreign material present in the joint is destroyed, it must be borne in mind that they have the potential to contribute to the pathogenesis of the disease by damaging surrounding tissues. In this chapter, the PMNL will be reviewed with special emphasis on the cellular cytotoxic and degradative mechanisms which are employed in the course of combating the infection and their potential to damage components of the joint.

PMNL ORIGINS AND MATURATION

Maturation from pluripotent stem cell to mature PMNL takes about 14 days and can be divided into two stages, the mitotic stage and the postmitotic stage. During the mitotic stage, the PMNL precursors divide and granules containing stored lysosomal enzymes and other antimicrobial compounds are synthesized[4,5]. The azurophilic granules (so called because of their azure colour after treatment with Wright–Giemsa stain) are produced first. After their formation, the specific

136

granules are synthesized and, in the mature PMNL, these granules outnumber azurophilic by approximately two to one.

During the postmitotic phase, cells undergo maturation of the formed granules and protein synthesis ceases; nuclear chromatin becomes tight and rough endoplasmic reticulum virtually disappears. Also, the number of mitochondria present in each cell is reduced and glycolysis becomes the primary energy source. This cellular adaptation is important for later possible operation in situations where the oxygen tension is low, a condition which is found at inflammatory foci. As maturation proceeds, PMNL precursors acquire functional capabilities, such as the ability to phagocytose and respond to chemotactic stimuli[6,7]. On completion of maturation, the cells are fully formed, able to phagocytose and to kill invading micro-organisms, and, as such, are highly specialized end cells, incapable of further cell division or of major protein synthesis.

MARGINATION AND CHEMOTAXIS

Mature PMNL are released into the blood stream[8] at a rate of about 110 billion cells per day. To maintain such a rate of release, the production of cells must be commensurately large. It is not surprising that 50% of the cells in the bone marrow at any one time are mature PMNL or their precursors. The pool of mature cells in the bone marrow awaiting release is thirty times larger than the pool of circulating PMNL and can be mobilized rapidly in response to an infection. Once in the bloodstream, PMNL have a circulation half-life of six to seven hours. The cells then marginate into the tissues where they may exist for one to four days. The actual length of time is unknown, as the tracing of PMNL in living tissues is a very difficult procedure[9].

Margination is the process of PMNL leaving the blood stream and entering the tissues. PMNL leave the capillary endothelium via the interendothelial cell junctions[10]. The process involves the degranulation of specific granules, presumably to allow the cell to digest its way through the junction. This does not appear to inflict permanent damage on the junction[11]. Also, the specific granular membranes are storage sites of C3 receptors and other substances, such as cytochrome b$_{-245}$, which are incorporated into the plasma membrane on degranu-lation[12]. Such incorporation might be important in priming the cell prior to chemotaxis and phagocytosis.

It is probable that margination is stimulated by localized inflam-mation caused by the presence of live micro-organisms or foreign anti-gen in the joint. Such foreign surfaces might activate complement and local cell damage would release other inflammatory mediators, such as prostaglandins and leukotrienes.

After margination, PMNL orientate themselves along the chem-otactic gradient formed by chemotactic factors and move towards the source of attractant. The cell assumes an internal asymmetry with the nucleus at the rear of the cell, the granule containing cytoplasm in the middle and microtubule array and pseudopods at the cell migration front[13–15]. Chemotactic factors are a heterogeneous group and include complement degradation fragments such as C5a[16] and derivatives of arachidonic acid generated by lipoxygenase and cyclo-oxygenase pathways[17].

.

PHAGOCYTOSIS

PMNL enter the joint space and move up the chemotactic gradient towards the source of the attractant and phagocytosis commences. Phagocytosis is a complex process involving the encapsulation and destruction of the micro-organism.

Destruction is achieved using two mechanisms, namely reactive oxygen species (ROS) and lysosomal enzyme release. Production of ROS commences within seconds of contact with the target and involves the production of molecules such as superoxide radical and oxygen halide ions. Ectoplasmic processes extend from the plasma membrane and gradually engulf the target; as this occurs, granules within the cell move towards the area of the plasma membrane in contact with the target, eventually fusing with, and then degranulating into, the forming phagocytic vacuole. Since the granule contents are not released into sealed phagolysosomes, there is leakage into the extra-cellular medium[18], determined by the size of the particle being phag-ocytosed and the availability of plasma membrane. This leakage might be copious, for example during the phagocytosis of large particles

138

such as MSU crystals or large aggregates of immune complexes. Also, there can be fusion of granules with plasma membrane which has not been stimulated or been in contact with a particle but with soluble stimuli. This is termed 'secretion'[19]. In addition, 'reverse endocytosis' or 'frustrated phagocytosis' could occur, where PMNL discharge their granules onto immune complexes attached to solid surfaces[20]. Thus, there is the potential for considerable local tissue damage and the exacerbation of the existing inflammation by constituents released from activated PMNL in the course of their normal function as they phagocytose infecting micro-organisms or immune complexes.

Reactive oxygen species

In 1933, Baldridge and Gerard[21] observed that granulocytes substantially increased their oxygen consumption on commencing phagocytosis. Generally it was thought that this was a result of phagocytosis being an active process. However, over 20 years later, it was discovered that increased oxygen consumption was accompanied by increased glucose catabolism via the hexose monophosphate shunt (HMPS). These two coinciding events which occur on activation of phagocytes have been termed the respiratory burst. Oxygen consumption of PMNL can increase by a factor of 40 as the cell produces superoxide radicals. Research into the production of superoxide and the other ROS produced by phagocytes has been an area of intense interest in the last one and a half decades and has revealed that ROS play a central role in PMNL cytotoxic mechanisms (for reviews see references 22–25). Moreover, ROS appear to be involved in the activation of enzymes and also act as inflammatory mediators.

Central to the production of ROS is the enzyme complex NADPH oxidase which is located in the plasma membrane of the PMNL. The enzyme catalyses the reduction of dioxygen to superoxide using reduced nicotinamide adenine dinucleotide phosphate, produced from the HMPS:

$$12NADPH + 24O_2 \rightarrow 24O_2^{\cdot -} + 12NADP^+ + 12H^+$$

This complex consists of a cytochrome, cytochrome b_{-245} which is unique to phagocytes[26], a FAD flavoprotein[27] and possibly ubiquinone[28]. Defects in this enzyme and subsequent defects in bacterial killing by PMNL are observed in patients with chronic granulomatous disease. This very rare disease has highlighted the central role played by ROS in PMNL cytotoxic mechanisms.

Orientation studies have shown that the enzyme produces super-oxide radical at the site of contact with the stimulus and superoxide-producing enzyme is located in the part of the plasma membrane which forms the phagocytic vacuole[29].

The superoxide radical is not a violent reagent. It can act as a nucleotide in hydrophobic environments and attack groups such as ester–carbonyl groups associated with phospholipids. Thus, it is poss-ible that the radical could damage synovial cells by membrane dis-ruption during phagocytosis by PMNL, especially if such phagocytosis was conducted on the synovium or very close to it. Studies indicate that the radical is capable of damaging biological materials[30,31], including glutathione peroxidase, an enzyme involved in PMNL radical defence[32]. However, 80% of the superoxide produced by PMNL is converted into hydrogen peroxide[33].

The addition of a second electron to superoxide results in the formation of the peroxide ion; peroxide formed at physiological pH immediately protonates to give hydrogen peroxide[34]. The overall reac-tion can be expressed as follows:

$$2O_2^{\cdot-} + 2H^+ \rightarrow H_2O_2 + O_2$$

The rate of dismutation increases as the pH decreases: thus, it is probable that, as the phagolysosome forms, the rate of hydrogen peroxide production increases since the pH within the phagolysosome decreases during formation.

Hydrogen peroxide is known to be toxic to bacteria and mammalian cells[35]. However, the major fate of hydrogen peroxide is the production of oxygen halide ions produced by the enzyme, myeloperoxidase. This enzyme is a 150 kDa glycoprotein stored in the azurophilic granules and constitutes 5% of the PMNL dry weight[36]. Its function in microbial killing has been extensively scrutinized since it was shown that the purified enzyme, hydrogen peroxide and chloride ions produced a highly potent antimicrobial agent[37]. The enzyme is capable of reacting with other halides but chloride ion is the preferred sub-strate[38,39]. The enzyme catalyses the oxidation of chloride in forming hypochlorous acid:

$$H_2O_2 + Cl^- + H^+ \rightarrow HOCl + H_2O$$

The pK_a of hypochlorous acid is 7.5; thus, at physiological pH, the acid is in approximate equilibrium with its dissociated form, the hypochlorite ion.

Potentially, hypochlorous acid can react in a number of different ways, including reaction with further chloride ions to form chlorine and decarboxylation reactions with amino acids[40]. However, the most potent form of reaction is thought to be with low molecular weight amines to form chloramines:

$$R-NH_2 + HOCl \rightarrow R-NHCl + H_2O$$

Two types of chloramine can be formed: the long-life type react with sulphydryl or thioester bonds[41]; the highly toxic type, which is lipophilic, is involved in membrane damage[42]. Other mechanisms by which this system may kill bacteria include the production of bactericidal aldehydes generated from free amino acids and the decaboxylation of amino acids in bacterial cell walls, resulting in peptide cleavage and subsequent loss of cell wall integrity[23]. Although the above reactions are targetted at the object being phagocytosed, there is considerable scope for such reactions damaging joint tissues in the locality of the phagocytosing PMNL.

Other ROS which could be produced include the hydroxyl radical which could be produced by two possible routes. The first route is the Haber–Weiss reaction, where superoxide and hydrogen peroxide react to form the hydroxyl radical:

$$O_2^{\cdot -} + H_2O_2 \rightarrow OH^{\cdot} + OH^- + O_2$$

However, kinetic studies in aqueous solutions suggest that the rate constant is very low. Also, it is unlikely that the concentrations of reagents are high enough for the reaction to occur *in vivo*.

The second reaction, which is kinetically more favourable, is the superoxide-driven Fenton reaction:

$$Fe^{3+} + O_2^{\cdot -} \rightarrow Fe^{2+} + O_2$$
$$\underline{Fe^{2+} + H_2O_2 \rightarrow Fe^{3+} + OH^- + OH^{\cdot}}$$

$$O_2^{\cdot -} + H_2O_2 \rightarrow O_2 + OH^- + OH^{\cdot}$$

141

This reaction requires a free iron co-ordination site[43,44]. Catalysis of the reaction may occur with copper and manganese. Iron is available in certain scenarios for the possible catalysis of the reaction; sufficient levels (μmol/L) are present in inflammatory exudates and rheumatoid arthritis synovial fluid samples[34]. Also, several types of micro-organisms have sufficient iron present in a usable form for catalysis. It should be stressed that levels of free iron in biology are normally zero; most of the iron in the human body is complexed to proteins, nucleic acids, phospholipids or low molecular weight chelating agents, such as citrate, ascorbate or ATP. Although chelated iron could possibly participate in such a reaction, this pool of iron is very small[34]. Experiments to ascertain whether the radical is produced in the course of PMNL function have so far proved inconclusive because chemical studies and electron spin resonance trap methods have proved to be too insensitive or non-specific to detect the radical[43].

This radical is a particularly attractive candidate since it is highly reactive, capable of initiating lipid peroxidation and addition onto aromatic ring structures.

The singlet oxygen radical also could be produced by activated PMNL though this is now thought to be unlikely because of the reaction rates, availability of reagents and pH considerations[35].

The potential for damage to joint components by ROS is considerable and there is abundant evidence to implicate these molecules in mediating tissue injury *in vivo*. PMNL phagocytosing foreign substances on the surfaces of the synovial membrane or articular cartilage would leak ROS from forming phagolysosomes. Possible membrane damage to chondrocytes and synovial cells by such species includes secondary radical formation within the membrane, lipid peroxidation and damage to membrane glycoproteins by oxidation[25].

Also these species can alter the biochemical and biophysical properties of structural proteins, including collagen and elastin[44-46]. Incubation of hyaluronic acid with superoxide and hydrogen peroxide generating systems alters the molecule, resulting in decreased viscosity and increased digestion by N-acetyl-β-D-glucosaminidase[47]. ROS damage to macromolecules is likely to render them more susceptible to protease and acid hydrolase degradation. Thus, it is possible that ROS and lysosomal enzymes act in concert to initiate tissue injury and further promote the acute inflammatory response.

ENZYME RELEASE

There are at least three types of granules in the human PMNL[19]. These are the azurophilic, specific and tertiary granules. The latter type are an ill-defined group, consisting of a range of smaller storage particles. A list of the enzymes contained within the azurophilic granule is presented in Table 9.1; it is an impressive list which can be divided into four sections: microbicidal enzymes, neutral proteinases, acid hydrolases and other proteins.

The microbicidal enzymes consist of myeloperoxidase (see section above) and lysozyme, which is a 14 kDa protein; it is a heat-stable cationic protein which attacks specifically the β-1–4 glycosidic linkage which joins N-acetyl muramic acid and N-acetyl glucosamine in the murein back-bone of peptidoglycan, present in bacterial cell walls[48]. Although this enzyme is specific for bacterial cell walls, there are a number of species which are resistant to its action, including group A streptococcus, staphylococci and almost all Gram-negative bacteria[49].

TABLE 9.1   Known constituents of human PMNL granules (adapted from references 19 and 65)

Azurophilic granules	Specific granules	Tertiary granules
Collagenase	Collagenase	Gelatinase
Elastase		Proteinase 3
Proteinase 3		
Cathepsin G		
Cathepsin B and D	Receptors for FMLP	Cathepsin B and D
β-Glucuronidase	C3bi receptors	β-Glucuronidase
β-Glycerophosphatase	Cytochrome b$_{-245}$	β-Glycerophosphatase
α-Mannosidase		α-Mannosidase
N-acetyl-β-glucosaminidase		N-acetyl-β-glucosaminidase
Ribonuclease		
Deoxyribonuclease		
Lysozyme	Lysozyme	
Myeloperoxidase	Vitamin B$_{12}$-binding protein	
Antimicrobial	Lactoferrin	
Cationic proteins	Complement activator	

It appears that the enzyme can still attack these targets if they are 'sensitized' by pretreatment with other factors; these include the serum antibody–complement system[50], a combination of ascorbate and hydrogen peroxide[51], antibiotics against cell walls and proteases[52]. Thus, it appears that lysozyme acts in concert with other cellular processes to destroy bacteria, since many of the clinically significant types are resistant to its action alone. Indeed, the main function of this enzyme may be the digestion of dead bacteria, killed by other cellular mechanisms[49].

The neutral proteinases contained within the azurophil granule have been categorized into three different types: elastase, cathepsin G and proteinase 3.

Elastase, a serine protease, is a 33–36 kDa molecular weight glycoprotein; at least three isoenzymes are present, differing in their carbohydrate content; these are believed to be present in various subpopulations of primary granules[53]. The enzyme is optimally active around pH 7.0 and can degrade macromolecules, such as collagen, elastin, proteoglycans, fibrinogen and fibronectin; it also cleaves immunoglobulins and complement[54].

The enzyme is very potent and is inhibited by acute-phase proteins circulating in the plasma and in the inflammatory exudate, such as α_1-antitrypsin and α_2-macroglobulin[55]. Indeed, the production of acute-phase proteins by the liver and cells in the locality of the inflammation increases dramatically and their binding to enzymes leaked by phagocytosing PMNL helps limit the damage to surrounding host tissue[56].

Studies suggest that elastase action is one of the major causes of PMNL-mediated endothelial cell injury[57] and is implicated in various diseases, including arthritis, cystic fibrosis and adult respiratory distress syndrome[58].

Cathepsin G acts on tyrosine and is a serine esterase; its natural substrates include cartilage proteoglycan, fibrinogen and complement. Like elastase, some of its cleavage products can act as chemotactic factors[54].

Proteinase 3 is distinguished from the above proteinases by its preference for the synthetic substrate, α-naphthyl acetate[59].

The known acid hydrolases present in the azurophilic granules constitute a formidable range of enzymes catalysing a wide range of reactions of a degradative nature.

144

Cathepsins B and D are acid proteinases which can be designated as thiol and carboxyl proteinases respectively[59]. The cathepsins are identified as different by the use of synthetic substrates[54].

The remaining enzymes in this particular group are polysaccharide and mucopolysaccharide hydrolysing enzymes. α-Mannosidase catalyses the removal of mannosides from sugar chains. N-acetyl-β-glucosaminidase cleaves glycosidic bonds adjacent to N-acetyl-β-glucosamine. β-Glucuronidase catalyses the hydrolysis of the glucuronidic bond at the non-reducing end of oligosaccharides[60].

A further group of proteins are found primarily in the azurophilic granules, termed cationic proteins[61]; this group seems to be a number of arginine-rich proteins, in the size range 10–25 kDa, which display antibacterial and antifungal activities[49]; these activities are non-enzymic. Part of this group consists of a collection of peptides, called defensins[62-64]. The peptides are 32–34 residues in length, with a common back-bone of eleven residues, and possess bactericidal, fungicidal and antiviral activity.

It can be seen that the above group of enzymes are bactericidal and essentially degradative. Thus, the azurophilic granules can be considered as being involved in bacterial killing and degradation[19,65].

Specific granules contain a different array of constituents from the azurophilic type (see Table 9.1). Lysozyme is found in this granule (see section above), along with the neutral proteinase, collagenase, and two particular binding proteins.

Collagenase is a 76 kDa protein, comprising two subunits of 42 and 33 kDa molecular weight[66]. The enzyme degrades type I collagen (most common in bone and tendon) and, at a lesser rate, type III collagen and appears to be resistant to inactivation by α_2-macroglobulin[67]. There is considerable evidence that the enzyme is stored in a latent form, termed procollagenase, and is activated by hypochlorous acid and, perhaps, directly by oxygen free radicals[68,69].

Lactoferrin is a 77 kDa protein which has a high affinity for iron[49]. It is stored in an unsaturated form and, on release, binds free iron which is essential for bacterial growth. The protein probably absorbs the free iron in the phagolysosome, hindering bacterial growth and possibly the generation of deleterious hydroxyl radical (see section above), though this latter point is disputed by some who consider that the lactoferrin iron would be available to participate in such radical generation[70]. In addition, lactoferrin inhibits the production of colony-stimulating factor from macrophages and increases PMNL adhesiveness[71].

Vitamin B_{12}-binding protein binds vitamin B_{12}, as the name implies, and is a requirement for bacterial growth. Thus, bacteria, during phagocytosis, are prevented from further growth and division in the forming phagolysosome. It is unlikely that the list above represents the full complement of the specific granule.

An important observation is that the granule membrane contains receptors for a variety of substances, suggesting that it forms some sort of store for the PMNL, which is unable to synthesize replacement receptors. C3bi receptors which are involved in phagocytosis have been reported[72,73], as have FMLP receptors[74]. It appears that the C3bi receptor may be involved in PMNL aggregation[65]. Also, there appears to be cytochrome b_{-245} present in the granule[75]. Complement activator and monocyte chemoattractant also are released from the specific granule[76,77]. Thus, specific granules contain a variety of constituents which reflect other functions of the granule like those seen during PMNL margination.

The tertiary granules in human PMNL are an ill-defined conglomerate of smaller storage particles. The structures contain predominantly cathepsins B and D, with some other acid hydrolases present (see Table 9.1). The only enzyme located solely in this granule type to date is gelatinase[78,79]. The enzyme, which cleaves collagen, is stored in a latent form and is activated by respiratory burst products[80].

The PMNL contains at least three different granule types, probably with subpopulations within each group. The azurophilic granule appears to be a classic lysosomal granule; the specific granule has several possible functions beyond just the bactericidal one, probably including enhancing cell response to chemotactic signals. The tertiary granules are ill defined and assignment of any particular specialized functional activity must await further clarification of the group.

INFLAMMATORY MEDIATORS

Membrane events on stimulation activate the enzyme phospholipase C, which, in conjunction with the diacylglycerol lipase, results in the production of arachidonic acid[81]. Also, this polyunsaturated fatty acid can be directly liberated from phospholipids by phospholipase A_2.

On liberation, the arachidonic acid is metabolized to a variety of compounds which have various functions, via cyclo-oxygenase, 5-lipoxygenase and 12- or 15-lipoxygenase pathways. Products from these pathways are released from PMNL and have a variety of inflammatory modulating effects.

The products of the cyclo-oxygenase pathway form the prosta-glandin and thromboxane series[82]. Certain products can cause increased vascular permeability and vasodilatation (prostaglandins E_1 and E_2 repectively). However, products have been shown to inhibit enzyme release from PMNL, suggesting that they have an anti-inflammatory role in limiting PMNL enzyme release[17]. This pathway is thought to be inhibited by non-steroidal anti-inflammatory drugs (NSAIDs), though, in PMNL, the drugs may have direct effects on their activation[83].

The lipoxygenase pathways produce leukotrienes (LT)[81,84]. On activation, human PMNL release into the surrounding medium a particularly potent leukotriene, B_4. This particular substance can cause chemotaxis, chemokinesis, aggregation, lysosomal enzyme release and superoxide generation from PMNL[81]. In addition, LTs C_4, D_4 and E_4 can be produced in different tissues depending on the enzymes present. The PMNL produces LTC_4, which can cause a variety of pro-inflammatory effects, including oedema, vasoconstriction and leakage from postcapillary venules[84].

CONCLUDING REMARKS

The PMNL play a central role in infective arthritis, phagocytosing and killing bacterial and fungal causative agents, and also removing and degrading antigen causing the acute inflammatory response observed in the infected joint.

Reactive oxygen species, including superoxide and oxygen halide

147

radicals and enzymes and other components released from the three granule types present in the PMNL provide a comprehensive group of killing and degradative mechanisms, capable of eradicating the infection. In addition, some of these may contribute to the inflammation observed during the course of its resolution.

REFERENCES

1. Platt, P. N. (1983). Examination of synovial fluid. In Dick, W. C. and Jeffery, M. S. (eds.) *Clinics in Rheumatic Diseases*, Vol. 9, No. 1, p. 54. (London: WB Saunders Co.)
2. Hurley, J. V. (1983). *Acute Inflammation,* 2nd Edn. (Edinburgh, London, Melborne and New York: Churchill Livingstone)
3. Ropes, M. W. and Bauer, W. (1953). *Synovial Fluid Changes in Joint Diseases.* (Cambridge MA: Harvard University Press)
4. Bainton, D. F., Ullyot, J. L. and Farquhar, M. G. (1971). The development of neutrophil polymorphonuclear leukocytes in human bone marrow. *J. Exp. Med.,* **134,** 907–934
5. Breton-Garius, R. and Reyes, F. (1976). Ultrastructure of human bone marrow maturation *Int. Rev. Cytol.,* **46,** 251–321
6. Lichtman, M. A. and Weed, R. I. (1970). Electrophoretic mobility and N-acetyl neuraminic acid content of human and leukemic lymphocytes and granulocytes. *Blood,* **35,** 12–22
7. Lichtman, M. A. and Weed, R. I. (1972). Alteration of the cell periphery during granulocyte maturation: relationship to cell function. *Blood,* **39,** 301–316
8. Mary, J. Y. (1985). Normal human granulopoiesis revisited. II. Bone marrow data. *Biomed. Biopharmacother.,* **39,** 66–77
9. Murphy, P. (1976). *The Neutrophil.* (New York and London: Plenum Medical Book Company)
10. Marchesi, V. T. (1961). The site of leucocyte emigration during inflammation. *Q. J. Exp. Physiol.,* **46,** 115–123
11. Marchesi, V. T. and Florey, H. W. (1960). Electron micrographic observation on the emigration of leucocytes *Q. J. Exp. Physiol.,* **45,** 343–348
12. Harlan, J. M. (1985). Leukocyte-endothelial reactions. *Blood,* **65,** 513–525
13. Ramsey, W. S. (1972). Analysis of individual leukocyte behaviour during chemotaxis. *Exp. Cell Res.,* **70,** 120–139
14. Ramsey, W. S. (1972). Locomotion of human polymorphonuclear leukocytes. *Exp. Cell Res.,* **72,** 489–500
15. Maleh, H. L., Root, R. K. and Gallin, J. I. (1977). Structural analysis of human neutrophil migration (centriole, microtubule and microfilament orientation and function during chemotaxis). *J. Cell Biol.,* **75,** 666–693
16. Chenoweth, D. E. and Hugli, T. E. (1978). Demonstration of a specific C5a receptor on intact human polymorphonuclear leukocytes. *Proc. Natl. Acad. Sci. USA,* **75,** 3943–3947
17. Abramson, S. and Weissmann, G. (1981). The release of inflammatory mediators from neutrophils. *La Ricerca Clin. Lab.,* **11,** 91–99

18. Weissmann, G., Korchak, H. M., Perez, H. D., Smolen, J. E., Goldstein, I. M. and Hoffstein, S. T. (1979). *J. Reticuloendothel. Soc.*, **26**, 687–700
19. Baggiolini, M. and Dewald, B. (1985). The neutrophil. *Int. Arch. Appl. Immunol.*, **76** (Suppl. 1), 13–20
20. Smolen, J. E. and Weissmann, G. (1979). Polymorphonuclear leukocytes. In McCarty, D. J. (ed.) *Arthritis and Allied Conditions: A Textbook of Rheumatology*, pp. 282–295. (Philadelphia: Lea and Febiger)
21. Baldridge, C. W. and Gerard, R. W. (1933). The extra respiration of phagocytes *Am. J. Physiol.*, **103**, 235–236
22. Fantone, J. C. and Ward, P. A. (1982). Role of oxygen derived free radicals and metabolites in leukocyte dependent inflammatory reactions. *Am. J. Pathol.*, **107**, 397–418
23. Beaman, L. and Beaman, B. L. (1984). The role of oxygen and its derivatives in microbial pathogenesis and host defense. *Annu. Rev. Microbiol.*, **38**, 27–48
24. Rossi, F., Bellavite, P., Berton, G., Grzeshowiak, M. and Papini, E. (1985). Mechanism of production of toxic oxygen radicals by granulocytes and their function in the inflammatory process. *Pathol. Res. Pract.*, **180**, 136–142
25. Fantone, J. C. and Ward, P. A. (1985). Polymorphonuclear leukocyte mediated cell and tissue injury: oxygen metabolites and their relation to human disease. *Human Pathol.*, **16**, 973–978
26. Hattori, H. (1961). Studies on the labile stable NADH oxidase and peroxidase staining reactions in the granulocyte particles of the horse granulocyte. *Nagoya J. Med. Sci.*, **23**, 362–378
27. Bellavite, P., Cross, A. R., Serra, M. C., Davoli, A., Jones, O. T. G. and Rossi, F. (1983). The cytochrome B and flavin content and properties of the superoxide forming NADPH oxidase solubilized from activated neutrophils. *Biochim. Biophys. Acta*, **746**, 40–47
28. Crawford, D. R. and Schneider, D. L. (1982). Identification of ubiquinone 50 in human neutrophils and its role in microbicidal events. *J. Biol. Chem.*, **257**, 6662–6668
29. Allen, R. C. (1982) Biochemiexcitation: chemiluminescence and the study of biological oxygenation reactions. In Deluca, M. A. and McElroy, W. D. (eds.) *Chemical and Biological Generation of Excited States*, pp. 309–344. (New York: Academic Press)
30. Halliwell, B. and Gutteridge, J. M. C. (1985). The importance of free radicals and the catalytic metal ions in human diseases. *Mol. Aspects Med.*, **8**, 89–193
31. Halliwell, B. and Gutteridge, J. M. C. (1985). *Free Radicals in Biology and Medicine*. (Oxford: Clarendon Press)
32. Blum, J. and Fridovich, I. (1985). Inactivation of glutathione peroxidase by superoxide radicals. *Arch. Biochem. Biophys.*, **240**, 500–508
33. Root, R. K., and Metcalf, J. A. (1977). H_2O_2 release from human granulocytes during phagocytosis: relationship to superoxide anion formation and cellular catabolism of H_2O_2: studies with normal and cytochalasin B treated cells. *J. Cell Invest.*, **60**, 1266–1276
34. Halliwell, B. and Gutteridge, J. M. C. (1984). Oxygen toxicity, oxygen radicals, transition metals and disease. *Biochem. J.*, **219**, 1–14
35. Klebanoff, S. J. (1982). Oxygen dependent cytotoxic mechanisms of phagocytes. In Gallin, J. I. and Fauci, A. S. (eds.) *Advances in Host Defence Mechanisms*, Vol. I. (New York: Raven Press)

36. Schultz, J. and Kaminker, K. (1962). Myeloperoxidase of the leucocytes of normal human blood. I. Content and localisation. *Arch. Biochem.*, **96**, 465–467
37. Klebanoff, S. J. (1968). Myeloperoxidase–halide–hydrogen peroxide antibacterial system. *J. Bacteriol.*, **95**, 2131–2138
38. Zgliczynski, J. M., Selvaraj, R. J., Paul, B. B., Stelmazynska, T, Poshitt, P. K. F. and Sbarra, A. J. (1977). Chlorination by the myeloperoxidase H_2O_2-Cl-antimicrobial system at acid and neutral pH. *Proc. Soc. Exp. Biol. Med.*, **154**, 418–422
39. Thomas, E. L. and Fishman, M. (1986). Oxidation of chloride and thiocynate by isolated leukocytes. *J. Biol. Chem.*, **261**, 9694–9701
40. Babior, B. M. (1978). Oxygen dependent microbial killing by phagocytes. *N. Engl. J. Med.*, **298**, 659–668
41. Weiss, S. J., Lampert, M. B. and Test, S. T. (1983). Long lived oxidants generated by human neutrophils. *Science*, **222**, 625–628
42. Grisham, M. B., Jefferson, M. M., Melton, D. F. and Thomas, E. L. (1984). Chlorination of endogenous amines by isolated neutrophils. *J. Biol. Chem.*, **259**, 10404–10413
43. Tauber, A. I. and Babior, B. M. (1985). Neutrophil oxygen reduction: the enzyme and the products. *Adv. Free Rad. Biol. Med.*, **1**, 265–307
44. Greenwald, R. A. and Moy, W. W. (1979). Inhibition of collagen gelatin by the action of superoxide radical. *Arthritis Rheum.*, **22**, 251–257
45. Carp, H. and Janoff, A. (1983). Modulation of inflammatory cell protease-tissue antiprotease interactions at sites of inflammation by leukocyte derived oxidants. In Weissmann, G. (ed.) *Advances in Inflammation Research*, Vol. 5, pp. 173–201. (New York: Raven Press)
46. Bates, E. J., Harper, G. S. and Lowther, D. A. (1984). Effect of oxygen derived reactive species on cartilage proteoglycan-hyaluronic aggregates. *Biochem. Int.*, **8**, 629–636
47. Greenwald, R. A. and Moy, W. W. (1980). Effect of oxygen derived free radicals on hyaluronic acid. *Arthritis Rheum.*, **23**, 455–461
48. Strominger, J. L. and Ghuysen, J. M. (1967). Mechanisms of enzymatic bacteriolysis. *Science*, **156**, 213–221
49. Root, R. K. and Cohen, M. S. (1981). The microbicidal mechanisms of human neutrophils and eosinophils. *Rev. Infect. Dis.*, **3**, 565–598
50. Wilson, L. A. and Spitznagel, J. K. (1968). Molecular and structural damage to *E. coli* produced by antibody, complement and lysozyme systems. *J. Bacteriol.*, **96**, 1339–1348
51. Miller, T. E. (1969). Killing and lysis of Gram negative bacteria through the synergistic effect of hydrogen peroxide, ascorbic acid and lysozyme. *J. Bacteriol.*, **98**, 949–995
52. Efrati, C., Sachs, T., Ne'eman, N, Lahov, M. and Ginsburg, J. (1976). The effect of leukocyte hydrolyases on bacteria. III. The combined effect of leukocyte lysozyme enzymic cocktails and penicillin on the lysis of Staphylcoccus aureus and group A Streptococci in vitro. *Inflammation*, **1**, 371–407
53. Garcia, R. C., Peterson, C. G. B., Segal, A. W. and Venge, P. (1985). Elastase in the different primary granules of the human neutrophil. *Biochem. Biophys. Res. Commun.*, **132**, 1130–1136
54. Klebanoff, S. J. and Clark, R. A. (1978). *The Neutrophil: Function and Clinical Perspectives.* (Amsterdam, New York and Oxford: North Holland)

150

55. Travis, J. and Salvesen, G. S. (1983). Human plasma proteinase inhibitors. *Annu. Rev. Biochem.*, **52**, 655–709
56. Carr, W. P. (1983). Acute phase proteins. In Dick, W. C. and Jeffery, M. S. (eds.) *Clinics in Rheumatic Diseases*, Vol. 9., pp. 227–239. (London: W. B. Saunders Co.)
57. Smedly, L. A., Tonneson, M. G., Sandhaus, R. A., Haslett, C., Guthrie, L. A., Johnston, R. B., Henson, P. M. and Worthen, G. S. (1986). Neutrophil mediated injury to endothelial cells. Enhancement by endotoxin and essential role of neutrophil elastase. *J. Clin. Invest.*, **77**, 1233–1243.
58. Janoff, A. (1985). Elastase in tissue injury. *Annu. Rev. Med.*, **36**, 207–216
59. Baggiolini, M., Bretz, U. and Dewald, B. (1978). Subcellular localization of granulocyte enzymes. In Havemann, K., and Janoff, A. (eds.) *Neutral Proteases of Human Polymorphonuclear Leukocytes*, pp. 3–17. (Baltimore, Munich: Urban and Schwarzenberg)
60. White, A., Handler, P. and Smith, E. L., (1964). *Principles of Biochemistry*, 3rd Edn. p. 774. (New York, Toronto, London: McGraw-Hill Book Company)
61. Ohlsson, K., Ohlsson, I. and Spitznagel, J. K. (1977). Localisation of chymotrypsin like cationic protein, collagenase and elastase in azurophilic granules of human neutrophilic polymorphonuclear leukocytes. *Hoppe Seylers Z. Physiol. Chem.*, **358**, 361–366
62. Selsted, M. E., Brown, D. M., Delange, R. J., Harwig, S. S. L., Ganz, T., Schilling, J. W. and Lehrer, R. I. (1985). Primary structure of six antimicrobial peptides of rabbit peritoneal neutrophils. *J. Biol. Chem.*, **260**, 4579–4584
63. Selsted, M. E., Harwig, S. S. L., Ganz, T., Schilling, J. W. and Lehrer, R. I. (1985). Primary structure of three human neutrophil defensins. *J. Clin. Invest.*, **76**, 1436–1439
64. Ganz, T., Selsted, M. E., Szklarek, D., Harwig, S. S. L., Daker, K., Bainton, D. F. and Lehrer, R. I. (1985). Defensins: natural peptide antibiotics of human neutrophils. *J. Clin. Invest.*, **76**,1427–1435
65. Gallin, J. I. (1985). Neutrophil specific granule deficiency. *Annu. Rev. Med.*, **36**, 263–274
66. Ohlsson, K. (1978). Purification and properties of granulocyte collagenase and elastase. In Havemann, K. and Janoff, A. (eds.) *Neutral Proteases of Human Polymorphonuclear Leukocytes*, pp. 89–101. (Baltimore and Munich: Urban and Schwarzenberg)
67. Hasty, K. A., Hibbs, M. S., Kang, A. H. and Mainardi, C. L. (1984). Heterogenity among human collagenases demonstrated by monoclonal antibody that selectively recognizes and inhibits human neutrophil collagenase. *J. Exp. Med.*, **159**, 1455–1463
68. Weiss, S. J., Peppin, G. J. Ortiz, X., Ragdale, J. and Test, S. T. (1955). Oxidative autoactivation of latent collagenase by human neutrophils. *Science*, **227**, 747–749
69. Burkhardt, H., Schwingel, M., Menninger, H., MaCartney, H. W. and Tschesche, T. (1986). Oxygen radicals as effectors of cartilage destruction. Direct degradative effect on matrix components and indirect action via activation of latent collagenase from polymorphonuclear leukocytes. *Arthritis Rheum.*, **29**, 379–387
70. Ambrusco, D. R. and Johnston, R. B., (1981). Lactoferrin enhances hydroxyl radical production by human neutrophils, neutrophil particulate fractions and an enzymatic generating system. *J. Clin. Invest.*, **67**, 352–360

71. Boxer, L., Bjorksten, B., Bjork, J., Yang, H., Allen, J. M. and Baehner, R. M. (1982). Neutropenia induced by systemic infusion of lactoferrin. *J. Lab. Clin. Med.*, **99**, 866–872

72. O'Shea, J., Seligmann, B., Gallin, J. I., Chused, T., Berger, M., Frank, M. and Brown, E. (1984). Distinct modulation of complement receptors on human neutrophils. *Fed. Proc.*, **43**, 1505

73. Arnaout, M. A., Spits, H., Terhorst, C., Pitt, J. and Todel, R. F. (1984). Deficiency of a leukocyte glycoprotein (LFA-1) in two patients with MO 1 deficiency: effects of cell activation on MO 1/LFA 1 surface expression on normal and deficient leukocytes. *J. Clin. Invest.*, **74**, 1291–1300

74. Fletcher, M. and Gallin, J. I. (1983). Human neutrophils contain an intracellular pool of putative receptors for the chemoattractant N-formyl-methionylleucylphenylalanine. *Blood*, **62**, 792–799

75. Borregaard, N., Heiple, J. M., Simons, E. and Clark, R. A., (1983). Subcellular localization of the b cytochrome component of the human neutrophil microbicidal oxidase: translocation during activation. *J. Cell Biol.*, **97**, 52–61

76. Wright, D. G. and Gallin, J. I. (1977). A functional separation of human neutrophil granules: generation of C5a by a specific granule product and inactivation of C5a by azurophil granule products. *J. Immunol.*, **119**, 1068–1076

77. Wright, D. G. and Greenwald, D. (1979). Increased motility and maturation of human blood monocytes stimulated by products released from neutrophil secondary granules. *Blood*, **54**, (Suppl 1.), 95a

78. Murphy, G., Bretz, U., Baggiolini, M. and Reynolds, J. J., (1980). The latent collagenase and gelatinase of human polymorphonuclear leukocytes. *Biochem. J.*, **192**, 517–525

79. Dewald, B., Bretz, U. and Baggiolini, M. (1982). Release of gelatinase from a novel secretory component of human neutrophils. *J. Clin. Invest.*, **70**, 518–525

80. Peppin, G. J. and Weiss, S. J. (1986). Activation of the endogenous metalloproteinase, gelatinase, by triggered human neutrophils. *Proc. Natl. Acad. Sci. USA*, **83**, 4322–4326

81. Davies, P., Bailey, P. J. and Goldenberg, M. M. (1984). The role of arachidonic acid oxygenation products in pain and inflammation. *Annu. Rev. Immunol.*, **2**, 335–357

82. Granstrom, E. (1984). The arachidonic acid cascade. The prostaglandins, thromboxanes and leukotrienes. *Inflammation*, **8**, S15–S25

83. Abramson, S., Edelson, H., Kaplan, H., Ludewig, R. and Weissmann, G. (1984). Inhibition of neutrophil activation by non-steroidal anti-inflammatory drugs. *Am. J. Med.*, **77**, 3–6

84. Piper, P. (1984). Formation and action of leukotrienes. *Physiol. Rev.*, **64**, 744–761

10

PRESENTATION OF BACTERIAL ANTIGENS TO T LYMPHOCYTES

J. A. GOODACRE

INTRODUCTION

T lymphocytes use specific receptors to recognize short linear peptide antigens associated with 'self' MHC-encoded molecules on the surface membranes of antigen presenting cells (APC). In comparison B lymphocytes bind specifically free antigen using cell surface immunoglobulin, and antibodies usually recognise configurational epitopes. Besides the recognition of antigen other signals, mediated by accessory molecules and cytokines, may be needed for T cell activation to occur. T lymphocytes can be divided into at least two major subsets on the basis of their function, namely helper T lymphocytes, which facilitate the differentiation of B lymphocytes into antibody-secreting cells, and cytotoxic T lymphocytes which lyse infected cells. Much controversy continues to surround the possible existence of suppressor T lymphocytes as a separate subset. The activation of antigen-specific helper T lymphocytes is a fundamental step in the induction of immune responses. Until recently the mechanisms of antigen presentation had been studied only using experimental protein antigens, such as ovalbumin, but there is now increasing interest in the induction of T lymphocyte responses to bacterial antigens. These mechanisms may be relevant in two ways to the pathogenesis of arthritis. Firstly, in infective arthritis bacteria may be isolated from synovial fluid. The nature of the host's immune response to these bacteria at this site is likely to be important in determining the outcome of the disease and might also be important in determining initially the localization of infection to the joint. Secondly, the pathogenesis of chronic poly-arthritis (such as rheumatoid arthritis and ankylosing spondylitis) may be associated with bacterial infection. One mechanism for this might be that chronic polyarthritis results from the activation of T lymphocytes recognizing bacterial antigens which are hom-ologous to certain self proteins. These T lymphocytes might then induce cross-reactive immune responses to host tissue. The strongest evidence for this mechanism is that cloned T lymphocytes which recognize a defined antigen of *Mycobacterium tuberculosis* induce arthritis when injected into susceptible rats[1].

In this chapter the basic mechanisms of antigen presentation will be outlined and related to mechanisms of induction of T lymphocyte responses to bacterial antigens. Particular attention will be paid to the presentation and recognition of *M. tuberculosis* because of the known involvement of this bacterium in the pathogenesis of arthritis.

THE STRUCTURE AND FUNCTION OF THE MAJOR HISTOCOMPATIBILITY COMPLEX

A genetic component in the control of immune responses was first suggested by German physicians who noted that the outcome of diphtheria infection varied among different families. The importance of the Major Histocompatibility Complex (MHC) in the control of immune responses was first appreciated from studying mechanisms of graft rejection[2]. The availability of inbred strains of mice enabled the magnitude of graft rejection to be ascribed to differences between donor and recipient at loci at and within their MHC regions. MHC loci were divided into class I and II, the latter controlling the strongest rejection responses. Later, the control of the magnitude of responses to experimental protein antigens was mapped also to the MHC class II loci. It was suggested that the magnitude of immune responses was either mediated through direct involvement of MHC-encoded molecules in antigen recognition or through some constraint upon T lymphocytes, involving either the absence of T lymphocytes with the appropriate specificity or the action of suppressor T lymphocytes. There is evidence to support each of these models and the relative importance of each remains a subject for debate.

The human MHC, known as the HLA region, is found on chromosome six. Although analogous to murine MHC there are some differences in its structure and in particular the region encoding class II molecules is more complex[3]. There are at least three class II loci, called DP, DQ and DR (mice have only two) each of which contains genes encoding α and β chains of class II molecules. There are three class I loci, called B, C and A, separated from class II genes by a class III region which includes genes encoding for the complement components C2 and C4.

MHC MOLECULES AND THEIR INTERACTION WITH PEPTIDE ANTIGENS

MHC class I molecules comprise a single transmembrane glycoprotein, called the α chain, which is bound non-covalently to β_2-microglobulin[4]. All nucleated cells express class I molecules. MHC class II molecules comprise two transmembrane glycoproteins of similar molecular mass called the α and β chains[5]. These molecules have a more limited tissue distribution and are normally expressed only on dendritic cells (and related cell types), thymic epithelium, and some macrophages, B and (in humans) T lymphocytes. Many non-lymphoid cell types can be induced to express MHC class II, for example, by culturing with γ-interferon. Generally, cytotoxic T lymphocytes recognize antigens in association with MHC class I molecules whereas helper T lymphocytes recognize antigens in association with MHC class II molecules.

Following the demonstration that T lymphocytes have to recognize both antigen and 'self' MHC molecules[6,7] the question arose as to whether or not this was achieved using a single T cell receptor. Elegant experiments by Schwartz and co-workers[8] showed that the fine specificity of a peptide antigen from pigeon cytochrome c was determined by the MHC class II haplotype of the APC, suggesting that interaction between antigen and MHC class II molecules occurred. Then, Unanue and co-workers demonstrated, by equilibrium dialysis, binding in solution of a hen egg lysozyme peptide to purified MHC class II molecules from a responder, but not non-responder, haplotype[9]. Finally, Grey and co-workers used gel filtration to measure the rate

155

of binding of a variety of peptide antigens to purified MHC class II molecules[10]. Rates of association and dissociation were slow (relative to the rate of binding of antigens to antibodies) and the complexes were sufficiently stable to be presented in liposomes to antigen-specific T cell clones. These experiments showed that peptide antigens bind specifically to MHC molecules. Furthermore, the isolation and characterization of the genes encoding the α and β chains of the T cell receptor was followed by the demonstration that transfection of T cell receptor genes conferred upon the recipient T cell both the antigenic specificity and MHC restriction of the donor T cell[11]. Thus, there is strong evidence that antigen presentation is effected by a complex of peptide antigen bound to MHC molecule which is recognized by a single T cell receptor.

Much current interest is focused upon the configuration adopted *in situ* by peptide antigens in relation to the MHC molecule and T cell receptor. Some experiments suggest an α-helical[12], others a linear configuration[13], but there is no apparent reason why constraints on the options available should necessarily exist. Recently the crystal structure of an HLA class I molecule was elucidated[14] and from this a prediction of the tertiary structure of a class II molecule made[15]. The antigen binding region was formed by a groove distal to the cell membrane and comprised two α-helical structures each on either side of a floor formed by a β-pleated sheet. Although data on the three-dimensional structure of MHC molecules is limited at present, much of the available information is consistent with previous analyses identifying sites of polymorphism between, and sites of binding of alloantibodies to, MHC molecules.

Recently, strategies have been developed for predicting, on the basis of primary sequence, regions in proteins most likely to be antigenic for T lymphocytes. One approach was to identify sequences liable to form amphipathic α-helices in solution[16]. Another was based upon the identification of a characteristic 'motif' in approximately 80% of defined T cell epitopes which allowed prediction not only of the site of T cell epitopes but also of the MHC haplotype to which they would be restricted[17]. Analysis of a larger number of protein antigens will allow the general usefulness of these approaches to become clear.

ACCESSORY MOLECULES

In addition to the structures described above, which are concerned with specific recognition, other molecules on the APC and T lymphocyte are required in some cases for helper T cell activation. These include LFA-1[18], LFA-3[19], CD2[20] and CD4[21]. It appears that these molecules serve to promote cell–cell binding although knowledge of their function is incomplete. Similarly, cytokines such as IL-1[22] and IL-6[23] may have a role in activation of some T cells either through direct binding to the T lymphocyte or through an effect on the APC involved.

ANTIGEN PROCESSING

Proteins which contain antigens recognized by T lymphocytes often require structural alteration in order that the antigen may be presented. Early work showed that bacteria and experimental proteins were taken up and degraded by macrophages following which the antigens could be presented[24]. Furthermore, APC rendered metabolically inactive by fixation in glutaraldehyde could present degraded fragments of ovalbumin but not the native molecule to ovalbumin-specific T cell hybridomas[25]. Later, it was found that other pathways of processing existed besides that of intracellular degradation. Fixed APC could not present native myoglobin but did so when the myoglobin was methylated, a procedure which was thought to expose the T cell epitope by inducing conformational change in the molecule[26]. Some workers proposed a role for membrane-bound proteases in protein degradation[27], whilst others showed that native proteins could be presented in liposomes presumably because T cell epitopes were already exposed[28]. There has also been a broadening view of the types of cells capable of processing antigens. Macrophages are probably of particular importance for protein degradation, particularly for bacterial and experimental antigens, but non-phagocytic dendritic cells and B lymphocytes can also process some microbial antigens and the existence of class I-restricted cytotoxic T lymphocytes which recognize influenza virus nucleoprotein suggests that many types of target cell can process viruses to present internal viral antigens on their cell surface membranes[29].

ANTIGEN PRESENTING CELLS

Whilst early studies focused upon the role of macrophages it is now clear that other bone-marrow derived cell types are important APC. The functional significance of APC heterogeneity is not fully understood but there are known differences both in the ability of different APC to process and present different antigens, and in the types of T cells activated by different APC. Any cell which expresses MHC class II molecules has the potential to present antigen. Several non-myeloid cell types (such as endothelial cells[30]) have been induced to express MHC class II molecules *in vitro* and thus to function as APC for T cell lines or clones. However, the activation requirements of these highly-differentiated T cells are probably quite different from those of less-differentiated T cell populations, and it is questionable whether non-myeloid cells are important APC *in vivo*.

Steinman–Cohn Dendritic Cells

Dendritic cells (DC) were purified originally from mouse lymphoid tissues[31] and possess a characteristic dendritic morphology *in vitro*. They are non-phagocytic, transiently adherent cells which express a high density of MHC class II molecules on their surface membranes. They are potent cells for inducing syngeneic and allogeneic mixed leukocyte responses and can present experimental protein antigens, haptens, autoantigens and microbial antigens[32]. The ability of DC to present some microbial antigens is dependent upon the function of macrophages[33], perhaps indicating a limitation in their processing capacity. DC may be the most important APC for inducing primary T cell responses and the observation that they can present haptens to unprimed T lymphocytes is consistent with this view[34]. DC appear to be related closely to Langerhans cells, veiled cells and interdigitating cells (see below) and it seems likely that these cells are all the same type assuming slightly different phenotypes in different sites of the body. Cells with features similar to DC have been isolated from human peripheral blood and from sites of chronic inflammation, such as synovial fluid[35].

Langerhans Cells

Langerhans cells are found in mammalian epidermis where they have a dendritic morphology and express MHC class II molecules in large density. Langerhans cells contain characteristic intracellular organelles called Birbeck granules[36] whose function is unknown, and in humans express CD1 molecules on their cell surfaces[37]. It has been difficult to purify Langerhans cells from epidermis but they appear to be mobile cells and to have a central role in the induction of contact sensitization[34].

Veiled Cells

Veiled cells are found in afferent, but not efferent, lymphatics[38]. They are remarkably similar in phenotype and function to DC and are probably the form in which DC-like cells in the periphery, such as Langerhans cells, transport antigens to lymph nodes.

Interdigitating Cells

Interdigitating cells are dendritic cells seen in T cell areas of spleen and lymph node[39]. They are probably included in the populations purified as DC *in vitro*.

B Lymphocytes

B lymphocytes bind antigens specifically using cell membrane immunoglobulin receptors. Antigens may then be processed and T cell epitopes expressed in association with MHC class II molecules on B lymphocyte cell membranes[40]. This provides the basis for the delivery by T lymphocytes of help for antibody production. Antigen-specific helper T lymphocytes recognize and bind these complexes, subsequently delivering signals (such as cytokines) to facilitate differentiation of the B lymphocyte into an antibody-secreting cell. The T lymphocytes themselves may undergo proliferation subsequently. Although B lymphocytes are probably not required for the induction of primary T cell responses they appear to be important for the expansion of antigen-specific helper T lymphocyte populations *in vivo*.

Macrophages

Macrophages have a wide distribution in tissues and the circulation. They are adherent, phagocytic cells which have a variety of biological functions[41]. One characteristic is the presence of intracellular lysosomes which contain a variety of proteolytic enzymes. Macrophages either express or can be induced to express surface membrane MHC class II molecules. They are poor inducers of mixed leukocyte responses compared to DC and although they appear capable of presenting antigens to T lymphocytes it may be that their role as an antigen processing cell is more important.

T Lymphocytes

Some human T lymphocytes express MHC class II molecules. The general significance of this is unclear but it may provide a mechanism for presenting antigens from viruses which bind specifically to molecules expressed on T lymphocytes[42].

THE INDUCTION OF T LYMPHOCYTE RESPONSES TO BACTERIAL ANTIGENS

In the first definitive studies of antigen processing, presentation by macrophages of *Listeria monocytogenes* to MHC class II-restricted T cells was shown to be an active, time-dependent process involving an intracellular step[24]. After uptake of bacteria a period of sixty minutes was required before T lymphocytes would bind to the macrophages. This step was sensitive to treatment of macrophages with chloroquine or ammonium chloride, and after the stage of processing macrophages could be fixed in paraformaldehyde without abrogating their ability to present that antigen. Macrophages had also a critical role in the presentation of *Corynebacterium parvum* to specific T cell lines[33]. The ability of spleen DC to present these bacterial antigens was dependent upon the presence of macrophages, could not be reproduced by adding macrophage culture supernatant or IL-1 to the DC and was sensitive to treatment of the macrophages with chloroquine. In contrast, macrophages were not required for DC to present polymeric flagellar protein of *Salmonella*[33], purified protein derivative of *Mycobacterium tuberculosis*[43] or whole non-viable *M. tuberculosis* organisms[43]. Both DC and macrophages presented whole *Mycobacteria* but DC were more potent and their potency was not increased by the addition of macrophages. These experiments showed that phagocytic cells were not required for the presentation of antigens from whole *M. tuberculosis* and supported the view that DC can process bacterial proteins on their surface membranes.

THE ROLE OF T LYMPHOCYTE RESPONSES TO BACTERIAL ANTIGENS IN THE PATHOGENESIS OF CHRONIC POLYARTHRITIS

There are many recognized clinical associations between bacterial infections and the subsequent development of chronic, sometimes destructive, polyarthritis. One mechanism which could provide the basis for this association is that of immune cross-reactivity between bacterial antigens and host proteins. In susceptible strains of rats a single intradermal injection of complete Freund's adjuvant, containing killed *M. tuberculosis* in oil, induces chronic destructive arthritis which can be transferred to naive recipient rats by injection of lymphoid cells from affected rats. There may also be involvement of the spine, balanitis, urethritis, colitis, skin lesions and eye lesions[44]. This model can be reproduced using a variety of bacteria[45], including *Streptococci* (*mutans, pyogenes* and *mitis*), *Lactobacillus plantarum* and *Staphylococcus aureus*.

T lymphocytes were cloned from a cell line which responded *in vitro* to *M. tuberculosis*. Clone A2b induced arthritis when injected intravenously into irradiated rats whereas clone A2c protected against the induction of arthritis and induced remission in affected rats[1]. The results suggested that this model of chronic destructive arthritis was mediated by specific T lymphocytes but the mechanisms involved are unknown. Clones A2b and A2c had a similar, though not identical, fine specificity focused on residues 180–188 of a region within the 65 kD fraction of *M. tuberculosis*[46]. This region is homologous with *M. bovis* and is recognized also by human T lymphocytes. A comparative analysis of the 180–188 peptide revealed that four of the amino acids were identical to those within a nine amino acid sequence of rat proteoglycan link proteins. Link proteins are found close to where the core protein (from which different types of sugar chain extend) binds to the hyaluronic acid 'backbone' of the proteoglycan molecule. It was suggested that T lymphocytes specific for residues 180–188 of *M. tuberculosis* might cross-react with proteoglycan link proteins leading to the induction of chronic arthritis.

SUMMARY

There is increasing interest in the mechanisms by which bacterial antigens are processed and presented to helper T lymphocytes. These mechanisms are of fundamental importance for the induction of anti-body-mediated immunity. T cell responses to bacterial antigens may be important both in determining the outcome of infective arthritis and in the pathogenesis of chronic polyarthritis.

REFERENCES

1. Cohen, I. R., Holoshitz, J., van Eden, W. and Frenkel, A. (1985). T lymphocyte clones illuminate pathogenesis and affect therapy of experimental arthritis. *Arthritis Rheum.*, **28**, 841
2. Schwartz, R. H. (1986). Immune Response (Ir) genes of the murine Major Histocompatibility Complex. *Adv. Immunol.* 38, 31
3. De Vries, R. R. P. (1988). Immunogenetics: HLA and arthritis. In Goodacre, J. and Carson Dick, W. (eds) *Immunopathogenetic Mechanisms of Arthritis.* (Lancaster: MTP Press Ltd.)
4. Dobberstein, B., Kvist, S. and Roberts, L. (1982). Structure and biosynthesis of

162

histocompatibility antigens. *Phil. Trans. R. Soc. Lond.* **B300,** 161
 5. Kaufman, J. F., Auffray, C., Korman, A. J., Shackleford, D. A. and Strominger, J. (1984). The class II molecules of the human and murine Major Histocompatibility Complex. *Cell,* **36,** 1
 6. Rosenthal, A. S. and Shevach, E. M. (1973). Function of macrophages in antigen recognition by guinea pig T lymphocytes. I. Requirement for histocompatible macrophages and T lymphocytes. *J. Exp. Med.,* **138,** 1194.
 7. Zinkernagel, R. M. and Doherty, P. C. (1974). Antigen recognised by altered self. *Nature,* **248,** 701
 8. Heber-Katz, E., Schwartz, R. H., Matis, L. A., Hannum, C., Fairwell, T., Appella, E. and Hansburg, D. (1982). Contribution of antigen presenting cell major histocompatibility complex gene products to the specificity of antigen induced T cell activation. *J. Exp. Med.* **155,** 1086
 9. Babbitt, B. P., Allen, P., Matsueda, G., Haber, E. and Unanue, E. R. (1985). Binding of immunogenic peptides to Ia histocompatibility molecules. *Nature,* **317,** 359
10. Buus, S., Sette, A., Colon, S., Miles, C. and Grey, H. M. (1987). The relation between major histocompatibility complex (MHC) restriction and the capacity of Ia to bind immunogenic peptides. *Science,* **235,** 1353
11. Dembic, Z., Haas, W., Weiss, S., McCubrey, J., Kiefer, H., von Boehmer, H. and Steinmetz, M. (1986). Transfer of specificity by murine α and β T-cell receptor genes. *Nature* **320,** 232
12. Allen, P., Matsueda, G. R., Evans, R. J., Dunbar, J. B. Jr., Marshall, G. R. and Unanue, E. R. (1987). Identification of the T cell and Ia contact residues of a T cell antigenic epitope. *Nature,* **327,** 713
13. Sette, A., Buus, S., Colon, S., Smith, J. A., Miles, C. and Grey, H. M. (1987). Structural characteristics of an antigen required for its interaction with Ia and recognition by T cells. *Nature,* **328,** 395
14. Bjorkman, P. J., Saper, M. A., Samraoui, B., Bennett, W. S., Strominger, J. L. and Wiley, D. C. (1987). Structure of the human class I histocompatibility antigen, HLA-A2. *Nature,* **329,** 506
15. Brown, J. H., Jardetzky, T., Saper, M. A., Samraoui, B., Bjorkman, P. J. and Wiley, D. C. (1988). A hypothetical model of the foreign antigen binding site of class II histocompatibility molecules. *Nature,* **332,** 845
16. Delisi, C. and Berzofsky, J. A. (1985). T cell antigenic sites tend to be amphipathic structures *Proc. Natl. Acad. Sci. USA,* **82,** 7048
17. Rothbard, J. B. and Taylor, W. R. (1988). A sequence pattern common to T cell epitopes. *EMBO J.,* **7,** 93
18. Regnier-Vigouroux, A., Blanc, D., Pont, S., Marchetto, S. and Pierres, M. (1986). Accessory molecules and T cell activation. I. Antigen receptor avidity differentially influences T cell sensitivity to inhibition by monoclonal antibodies to LFA-1 and L3T4. *Eur. J. Immunol.,* **16,** 1385
19. Breitmeyer, J. B. (1987). How T cells communicate. *Nature,* **329,** 760
20. Meuer, S. C., Hussey, R. E., Fabbi, M., Fox, D. A., Acuto, O., Fitzgerald, K. A., Hodgson, J. C., Protentis, J. P., Schlossman, S. F. and Reinherz, E. L. (1984). An alternative pathway of T cell activation: a functional role for the 50 kd T11 sheep erythrocyte receptor protein *J. Exp. Med.,* **36,** 897
21. Saizawa, K., Rojo, J. and Janeway Jr, C. A. (1987). Evidence for a physical association of CD4 and CD3:α:β T cell receptor. *Nature,* **328,** 260

22. Dinarello, C. A., Cannon, J. G., Mier, J. W., Bernheim, H. A., Lopreste, G., Lynn, D. L., Love, R. N., Webb, A. C., Auron, P. E., Reuben, R. C., Rich, A., Wolff, S. M. and Putney, S. D. (1986). Multiple biological activities of human recombinant interleukin 1. *J. Clin. Invest.*,**77,** 1734

23. Houssiau, F. A., Coulie, P. G., Olive, D. and Van Snick, J. (1988). Synergistic activation of human T cells by interleukin 1 and interleukin 6. *Eur. J. Immunol.,* **18,** 653

24. Ziegler, H. J. and Unanue, E. R. (1981). Identification of a macrophage antigen processing event required for I-region restricted antigen presentation to T lymphocytes. *J. Immunol.,* **127,** 1869

25. Shimonkevitz, R., Kappler, J., Marrack, P. and Grey, H. (1983). Antigen recognition by H-2 restricted T cells. I. Cell-free antigen processing. *J. Exp. Med.,* **158,** 303

26. Streicher, H. Z., Berkower, I. J., Busch, M., Gurd, F. R. N. and Berzofsky, J. A. (1984). Antigen conformation determines processing requirements for cell activation. *Proc. Natl. Acad. Sci. USA.* **81,** 6831

27. Buus, S. and Werdelin, O. (1986). Oligopeptide antigens of the angiotensin lineage compete for presentation by paraformaldehyde-treated accessory cells to T cells. *J. Immunol.,* **136,** 459

28. Walden, P., Nagy, Z. A. and Klein, J. (1986). Antigen presentation by liposomes: inhibition with antibodies. *Eur. J. Immunol.,* **16,** 717

29. Townsend, A. E. M., Gotch, F. M. and Davey, J. (1985). Cytotoxic T cells recognize fragments of the influenza nucleoprotein. *Cell,* **42,** 457

30. Hirschberg, H., Bergh, O. J. and Thorsby, E. (1980). Antigen presenting properties of human vascular endothelial cells. *J. Exp. Med.,* **152,** 249

31. Steinman, R. M., and Cohn, Z. A. (1973). Identification of a novel cell type in peripheral lymphoid organs in mice. I. Morphology, quantitation, tissue distribution. *J. Exp. Med.,* **137,** 1142

32. Austyn, J. M. (1987). Lymphoid dendritic cells. *Immunology,* **62,** 161

33. Guidos, C., Sinha, A. A. and Lee K-C. (1987). Functional differences and complementation between dendritic cells and macrophages in T cell activation. *Immunology,* **61,** 269

34. Macatonia, S. E., Knight, S. C., Edwards, A. J., Griffiths, S. and Fryer, P. (1987). Localisation of antigen on lymph node dendritic cells following exposure to the contact sensitizer fluorescein isothiocyanate. *J. Exp. Med.* **166,** 1654

35. Harding, B. and Knight, S. C. (1986). The distribution of dendritic cells in the synovial fluids of patients with arthritis. *Clin. Exp. Immunol.,* **63,** 594

36. Birbeck, M. S., Breathnach, A. S. and Everall, J. D. (1961). An electron microscope study of basal melanocytes and high level clear cells (Langerhans cells) in vitiligo. *J. Invest. Dermatol.,* **37,** 51

37. Murphy, G. F., Bhan, A. K., Sato, S., Harrist, T. J. and Mihm, M. C. (1981). Characterisation of Langerhans cells by the use of monoclonal antibodies. *Lab. Invest.,* **45,** 465

38. Drexhage, H. A., Mullink, H., De Groot, J., Clarke, J. and Balfour, B. M. (1979). A study of cells present in peripheral lymph of pigs with special reference to a type of cell resembling the Langerhans cell. *Cell Tissue Res.,* **202,** 407

39. Kamperdijk, E. W. A., Kapsenberg, M. L., Van den Berg M. and Hoefsmit, E. C. M. (1985). Characterisation of dendritic cells isolated from normal and stimulated rat lymph nodes. *Cell Tissue Res.,* **242,** 469

40. Lanzavecchia, A. (1985). Antigen-specific interaction between T and B cells. *Nature*, **314**, 537
41. Unanue, E. R. (1972). The regulatory role of macrophages in antigenic stimulation. *Adv. Immunol.*, **15,** 95
42. Lanzavecchia, A., Roosnek, E., Gregory, T., Berman, P. and Abrignani, S. (1988). T cells can present antigens such as HIV gp120 targeted to their own surface molecules. *Nature*, **334,** 530
43. Kaye, P. M., Chain, B. M. and Feldmann, M. (1985). Non-phagocytic dendritic cells are effective accessory cells for anti-mycobacterial responses *in vitro*. *J. Immunol.*, **3,** 1930
44. Pearson, C. M. (1956). Development of arthritis, periarthritis and periostitis in rats given adjuvants. *Proc. Soc. Exp. Biol. Med.* **91,** 95
45. Ebringer, R. (1979). Spondylarthritis and the post-infectious syndromes. *Rheumatol. Rehab.*, **18,** 218
46. Van Eden W., Thole, J. E. R., van der Zee, R., Noordzij, A., van Embden, J. D. A., Hensen, E. J. and Cohen, I. R. (1988). Cloning of the mycobacterial epitope recognised by T lymphocytes in adjuvant arthritis. *Nature*, **331**, 171

INDEX

167